Board St

Transesophageal E

MW00851543

Board Stiff TEE

Transesophageal Echocardiography

Christopher J. Gallagher, MD

Assistant Professor
Department of Anesthesiology
University of Miami School of Medicine
Miami, Florida

Cover art and selected illustrations by J.C. Duffy

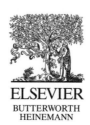

ELSEVIER
BUTTERWORTH
HEINEMANN

ELSEVIER
BUTTERWORTH
HEINEMANN

The Curtis Center
170 S Independence Mall W 300E
Philadelphia, Pennsylvania 19106

BOARD STIFF TEE: TRANSESOPHAGEAL ECHOCARDIOGRAPHY   0–7506–7515–2
Copyright © 2004, Elsevier Inc. All rights reserved.

No part of this publication may be reproduced or transmitted in any form or by any means, electronic or mechanical, including photocopying, recording, or any information storage and retrieval system, without permission in writing from the publisher. Permissions may be sought directly from Elsevier's Health Sciences Rights Department in Philadelphia, PA, USA: phone: (+1) 215 238 7869, fax: (+1) 215 238 2239, e-mail: healthpermissions@elsevier.com. You may also complete your request on-line via the Elsevier homepage (http://www.elsevier.com), by selecting 'Customer Support' and then 'Obtaining *Permissions*'.

NOTICE

Anesthesiology is an ever-changing field. Standard safety precautions must be followed but as new research and clinical experience broaden our knowledge, changes in treatment and drug therapy may become necessary or appropriate. Readers are advised to check the most current product information provided by the manufacturer of each drug to be administered to verify the recommended dose, the method and duration of administration, and contraindications. It is the responsibility of the treating physician, relying on experience and knowledge of the patient, to determine dosages and the best treatment for each individual patient. Neither the Publisher nor the author assumes any liability for any injury and/or damage to persons or property arising from this publication.

Every effort has been made to ensure that the drug dosage schedules within this text are accurate and conform to standards accepted at time of publication. However, as treatment recommendations vary in the light of continuing research and clinical experience, the reader is advised to verify drug dosage schedules herein with information found on product information sheets. This is especially true in cases of new or infrequently used drugs.

Recognizing the importance of preserving what has been written, Elsevier Inc. prints its books on acid-free paper whenever possible.

Library of Congress Cataloging-in-Publication Data

Gallagher, Christopher J.
  Board stiff TEE : transesophageal echocardiography / Christopher J. Gallagher.
    p. ; cm.
  Includes bibliographical references and index.
  ISBN 0–7506–7515–2
  1. Transesophageal echocardiography. I. Title: Transesophageal echocardiography. II. Title.
  [DNLM: 1. Echocardiography, Transesophageal—Examination Questions. 2. Echocardiography, Transesophageal—Resource Guides. WG 18.2 G162b 2004]
  RC683.5.T83G356 2004
  616.1'207543—dc22   2004045625

Printed in the United States of America

Last digit is the print number: 10   9   8   7   6   5   4   3   2   1

Dedication

To Guido, my bail bondsman.

Keep that cell phone on, Guido, you never know.

Preface

If you are doing cardiac anesthesia, cardiac surgery, or intensive care work, and you don't know Transesophageal Echocardiography, you are yesterday's newspaper. You are a repairman for 8-track cassette players. You are selling slide rules.

You need to know TEE.

Board Stiff TEE is just the ticket. I wrote this book to give you a complete introduction to the subject, from the physics of ultrasound to the images you need to recognize to the hemodynamic calculations you can make with TEE. The whole nine yards. Plus, I direct you to those places where you can deepen your understanding of TEE.

Board Stiff TEE is the perfect launch pad.

Board Stiff TEE is for the medical student, the anesthesiologist, the surgeon, the intensivist, who asks, "Just where do I start?"

The book details

- Why you need to know TEE
- Which books and meetings will help the most
- Everything you need to know if you take the PTEeXAM
- How to work through the quantitative aspects of TEE

Board Stiff TEE is jam-packed with simplified drawings to illustrate all the points you need to know. No need to decipher a small photograph of a TEE image; everything here is laid out with the student in mind. Especially when you start out, it's hard to tell what's what in a photograph of a TEE image. These drawings will lay it out for you.

Best of all, learning TEE does not have to be a replay of your root canal. *Board Stiff TEE* has a dollop of humor here and there to keep your eyes open and your airway from obstructing.

Several people helped in this affair. Alicia Borus gave expert secretarial help; my editor Natasha Andjelkovic reined in my more outlandish prose; Elsevier's illustrators redid all the drawings, improving on my "magic marker in a Crayola pad" work; and J.C. Duffy did the cover and the cartoons. Through it all, my wife endured my manic ravings.

And final thanks to my daughter Rachel, who is a blast.

Christopher J. Gallagher, MD

Acknowledgments

To Alicia Borus for secretarial expertise.

To my wife Carolyn, for enduring the unendurable— life with me.

To my daughter Rachel, for letting me use her Magic Markers to do the initial drawings for this monstrosity.

Contents

Introduction: Neither Rain nor Snow

The policeman tapped his baton on the bare foot sticking out of the refrigerator box. Behind the policeman, a mailman stood with his left hand on his leather satchel and his right hand holding a letter from the National Board of Echocardiography.

"Hey, rise and shine," the policeman said. "We have something for you, Dr. Gallagher."

Gray hair popped out of the other end of the refrigerator box. Gray hair disappearing in the middle, promising a "tonsured monk" look in another few years.

Eyes, rimmed red with hard living, hard anesthetizing, and bad investing, blinked in the sunshine just now peeking under the bridge.

"Officer!" the refrigerator box man said. "Why…" he looked around at the discarded MD 20/20 bottles wrapped in brown paper, the McDonald's bags, the metallic doo-dads that fell off passing cars. " … officer. Uh, excuse me while I freshen up."

The graying man pulled a Tony Roma's pre-moistened towelette packet out of his pocket, shook out a towlette, and rubbed some of the grime off his face.

"There," he wiggled out of the box, "now I'm presentable."

He stood up and brushed crumbs and critters off his green scrubs. On the front and back, large black lettering warned, "**Property of East Bumblebee Memorial Hospital. Rented, never sold.**"

The man looked down, then gave the policeman a sheepish grin.

"I'm renting."

"Uh-huh."

The mailman wrinkled his brow at that explanation, then lifted the envelope up to his face. "Says here, 'Dr. Chris Gallagher,' and for address it says, 'Under a bridge somewhere'." He looked up at the bridge, then down at the man in the scrubs. "Am I in the right place with the right person?"

"Why yes. Yes you are," the man in scrubs said. "I am, in point of fact, the very addressee you seek. It warms the cockles of my heart to see that, once again, 'Neither rain, nor snow, nor sleet, nor hail, nor heat of day, nor gloom of night, nor vagueness of address' have stayed you from the swift completion of your appointed rounds, my good mailperson."

Both policeman and mailman said, "Uh-huh."

Opening the letter, the man said, "Oh joy, rapture! I have passed the examination for special competence in the perioperative use of transesophageal echocardiography! Can you believe my good fortune?"

Policeman and mailman both shook their heads, apparently unable to believe the man's good fortune. Overhead, a big rig went "Thump!" and "Thump!" again as it roared over the expansion joints in the bridge.

The man in scrubs held his letter to his chest, right against the **"Property of East Bumblebee Memorial Hospital"** letters.

"Say," the man gave the policeman and mailman a conspiratorial look, "you don't suppose"—he looked behind lest someone surprise them, then turned back and stood on tiptoe to look over the shoulders of his two new friends—"you don't suppose I might parlay this little triumph into another book, do you?"

The policeman and mailman looked at each other.

"*Another* book?"

"Why yes," the man said. "A book about transesophageal echocardiography!"

"Who would want such a thing?" the policeman asked. He had served in the Miami Police Department for years. Talking with a babbling maniac was nothing new to him. At least *this* maniac wasn't shooting at anybody. The policeman preferred spending time with unarmed street people.

"Oh, anyone who might want to save a patient in hemodynamic trouble:

- Medical students

- ICU nurses

- Echocardiography technology students

- Anesthesiologists

- Anesthetists

- Intensivists of all flavors

- Cardiac surgeons

- ER and trauma center staff

- Anyone considering taking the Examination of Special Competence in Perioperative Transesophageal Echocardiography (PTEeXAM)."

"Thump! Thump!" "Thump! Thump!" Two more trucks passed overhead.

The mailman leaned on his left hip and shifted his leather satchel around. He had a few more letters to deliver, but didn't seem in a big rush.

The man in scrubs went on, "Transesophageal echocardiography is making its way into ICUs from sea to shining sea. It is THE way to diagnose hemodynamic instability in a hurry. A crystal ball looking into the near future shows TEEs appearing wherever and whenever a patient is crashing."

"And patients can crash anywhere!"

As if on cue, a driver on the bridge jammed on the brakes and a sickening squeal filled the air. All three men hunched their shoulders, squinted their eyes, and tensed for the "crash!"

But nothing happened. The policeman, mailman, and bescrubbed man all looked up, as if their eyes could pierce the concrete and figure out what happened.

Above, a string of obscenities in Spanish crackled in the air, then an engine roared to life and the car drove off.

"See what I mean?" the man said. "A crash can occur anywhere, anytime."

The policeman and mailman looked at each other and nodded. This nutcase was on to something here.

Reaching into the refrigerator box, the man in green scrubs pulled out a stack of papers, a sketch pad, and a magic marker.

"I'll throw together a little study guide from these notes I took. I'll include:

1. A guide to the books, meetings, and study material that will help you learn TEE.

2. A brief review for the Examination of Special Competence in Perioperative Transesophageal Echocardiography (PTEeXAM).

3. Detailed problem solving for the quantitative aspects of TEE, such as gradients, valve areas, and chamber pressures."

"For those of us who are visual learners," the mailman said, "do you feel that some simplified drawings may help out? Not that I anticipate much transesophageal echocardiography work at the Post Office, but you never know. Second careers and all that."

The man held up his magic marker. "Simplified drawings to aid the visual learner, coming right up."

1 · The Yellow Brick Road

"Follow the yellow brick road."

THE MAYOR OF MUNCHKINLAND
The Wizard of Oz

Dorothy received unambiguous directions to get where she needed to go. Here is your yellow brick road:

1. Go ye to the "Comprehensive Review of Intraoperative Echocardiography" meeting. It's held each year in February. For the next 5 years or so it will be held in San Diego. There are other echo meetings, including a quite similar review held in Atlanta in September every year. (The talks and speakers are similar at the meetings.) Both meetings are a little pricey but they are worth it! If you are considering taking the PTEeXAM, it's worth remembering that the same people who make up the exam give the lectures at the meeting. So figure it out, Sherlock. Need info? Go to the Society of Cardiovascular Anesthesiology Web site (*www.scahq.org*).

2. Do as much hands-on echo as you can at your hospital. Go to the echo lab. Ask if you can see some old tapes and go over them with a cardiologist. The more you DO, the more you LEARN.

3. Look at the content outline of the PTEeXAM and see if you know the subjects listed. That list is waiting for you at *www.echoboards.org/pte/pfoutline.html*.

4. Buy the complete set of tapes from the 2002 "Comprehensive Review" meeting. It's pricey (over a thousand smackers), and

lengthy (25 tapes, each about 2 hours long), but it's all there. Maybe get your department to buy a set of the tapes? Anyway, they are invaluable, full of great lectures, and all the TEE movies are reproduced clearly on the tapes. All in all, a good investment. Order them through CME Unlimited (phone: 800-776-5454 or 760-773-4498; fax: 760-773-9671; Web site: *www.CMEunlimited.org*).

5. If your pockets aren't that deep, buy the syllabuses from the meeting. There are two, one from days one through three of the meeting, and one from days four through six of the meeting. You can order them ($35 for one, $60 for the pair) from the Society of Cardiovascular Anesthesiology (phone: 804-282-0084; fax: 804-282-0090; E-mail: *sca@societyhq.com*; Web site: *www.scahq.org*). Tons of material from my studying and for this book came straight from those syllabuses.

6. Get ahold of the book most people use to study for the TEE exam, *Textbook of Clinical Echocardiography*, by Catherine M. Otto (W. B. Saunders, 2000; ISBN 0-7216-7669-3). When I talked to a sales representative at the TEE meeting in 2003, he confirmed what others told me—Otto has it all. (Between Otto and those syllabuses, you'll have all the "book reading" you could possibly need.)

7. Get the 2-CD set *TEE: An Interactive Board Review on CD-ROM*, edited by David S. Morse and C. David Collard (Lippincott Williams & Wilkins, 2002; ISBN 0-7817-3375-8). This has a series of TEE movies with attached tests. The tests are multiple choice (like the PTEeXAM). Once you've taken the test, you can check your answers. Best of all, each answer comes with a complete explanation along with references.

8. Another good CD is *TEE on CD: An Interactive Resource*, edited by Steven N. Konstadt and Navin C. Nanda (Lippincott Williams & Wilkins, 2001; ISBN 0-7817-2629-8). This CD *does have* a lot more text than the Morse and Collard CDs, and it is tough to scroll text for a long time on a computer.

9. More CDs? You bet. Since echo is a *moving* image, it makes sense to get CDs that show TEE images *moving*. Look on *amazon.com*; at last count, there are 30-something books on transesophageal echocardiography, lots with accompanying CDs. Robert Savage himself (a Big Kahuna in echo circles and organizer of the big TEE meeting) will have a big book coming out soon, so snap it up!

10. A great book fresh off the press and specifically made for transesophageal echocardiography is *A Practical Approach to*

Transesophageal Echocardiography, edited by A. C. Perrino and S. T. Reeves (Lippincott Williams & Wilkins, 2003; ISBN 0-7817-3638-2). The second editor of this book is a fellow who talked at the big TEE conference in San Diego, Dr. Scott T. Reeves. Great speaker! Funny stories! Knows how to get his point across crystal clear and that's just what he and his co-editors did in this book. (If you're short on dough, buy their book, put mine back on the shelf, and use the money you saved to buy a gyro. Then eat the gyro while you're reading Perrino and Reeves' book — but don't spill the cucumber sauce all over the pictures.)

What now?

You have a long path ahead of you. No lions and tigers and bears, but plenty of stuff to learn.

So do like Dorothy. Put one foot ahead of the other, keep those ruby slippers on tight, and follow the yellow brick road.

2 · To the End, Then Stop

"Where shall I begin, please your Majesty?"
"Begin at the beginning, ... and go on till you come to the end;
then stop."
Alice's Adventures in Wonderland

LEWIS CARROLL

Taking on TEE is a bit like trying to bite a beachball. Just where exactly do you sink your teeth in? Where can you get any purchase on this big thing?

One way is to go over the SCA content outline, and make sure you can talk a little about each subject listed. Be sure you can draw at least a *schematic* diagram of what they're talking about.

And so I did.

We start at the beginning.

I. Principles of Ultrasound

Nature of Ultrasound: Compression and Rarefaction

Ultrasound is sound waves propagated through a medium at a frequency above that which we can hear. Imaging depends on displaying the time required for an ultrasound pulse to go to a cardiac structure and return. We acoustically challenged humans only hear from 20 cycles/second to 20,000 cycles/second, or 20 kilohertz (named after the famous physicist and car-rental magnate).

Ultrasound starts at 20 kilohertz (20 kHz). For our medical imaging, the frequency used is between 1 and 20 megahertz (1 and 20 MHz). Take a look at our probe, and you'll see something like 5 or 7 MHz.

Keep in mind that sound, or ultrasound, must get propagated through a medium.

Jimi Hendrix blasted his guitar through the AIR at Woodstock. You blast your ultrasound through the TISSUE and FLUID with your TEE. Remember the ads when *Alien* came out? "In space, no one can hear you scream." That's right, there's nothing to propagate in a vacuum. There's no air for you to compress and rarefy.

Ultrasound does not propagate in air; this will be a recurring problem. Ultrasound only propagates through tissue and fluids.

Frequency, Wavelength, and Tissue Propagation Velocity

Note that *frequency* is the number of complete cycles per second, and *wavelength* is the distance from one corresponding area to the next (usually peak to peak). *Propagation velocity* is the wavelength × frequency.

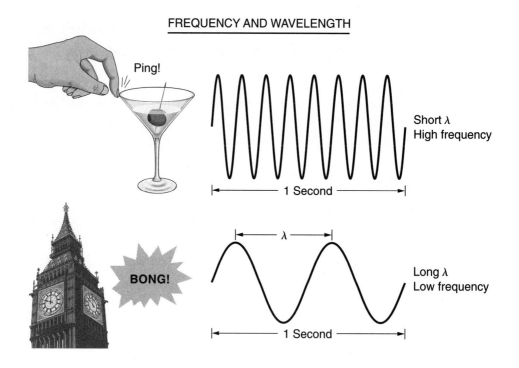

FREQUENCY AND WAVELENGTH

How does that relate to us? The propagation velocity of sound waves in human tissues is 1540 meters/second. So, since the velocity is pretty constant, that means the time it takes to go "out and back" correlates with distance. *Time is distance* is the basis of all "bounce technology" (sonar in a ship, locating enemy submarines; Doppler radar letting us know about a coming rainstorm; TEE telling us where the aortic dissection started).

Wavelength is important because resolution (the ability to tell two things apart) is no better than 1 or 2 wavelengths. So if you have a long, long wavelength, you won't be able to tell things apart very well. If you have a short, short wavelength, you *will* be able to tell tiny things apart. This comes into play when you are adjusting the wavelength for near and far objects.

A frequent consideration that occurs frequently with frequency is this: the higher the frequency, the better the resolution but the shallower the penetration.

The flip side, or the *wavelength paradigm*, is also true: the longer the wavelength, the deeper the penetration but the worse the resolution. The take-home message for budding TEE'ogists? To see an object close up, go to a higher frequency, and you'll see it in more detail. For a distant object — say, the pulmonic valve, which lies far from the TEE probe — use a longer wavelength (or, in other words, a lower frequency). This makes sense if you remember that frequency and wavelength are inversely related:

Up close: high frequency (or short wavelength)

Far away: low frequency (or long wavelength)

Properties of Ultrasound Waves

Ultrasound propagates poorly in a gas. That is the main property that concerns us, since, as you pull the probe higher and higher, you encounter the trachea or the left main bronchus getting between the probe and the heart. The gas in these structures forms an impenetrable (for ultrasound purposes) wall that obscures our vision, so we can't see parts of the aortic arch and the pulmonary arteries (we see the right for a while and a little of the left, but the left pulmonary artery, especially, gets "amputated" by the left mainstem bronchus).

This "air dilemma" also causes a problem with off-pump cases, in which the surgeon may hike the heart up and obscure your vision. (You need to retreat up the esophagus a little to get a view.)

Ultrasound–Tissue Interactions

Here's a little commonsense tip for ultrasound and tissue. Ultrasound in its usual diagnostic form doesn't hurt tissue. A zillion kids have been bombarded with ultrasound waves in utero, and, except for a fondness for MTV, bare midriffs, and pierced cartilage, there seems to have been no lasting damage. (Of course, cranked to the max, *sound* can crack stones, as we see in the ESWL suite every day.) But keep in mind that the probe is a machine that converts some of its energy to heat. So don't leave the probe running forever, lest you cause a burn to the esophagus. Turn the TEE off after you've done your study and let it cool.

Reflection   Ultrasound is based on reflection of the signal from internal structures. Ultrasound is reflected at tissue boundaries, and that is what allows us to see where, for example, the ventricle ends and the blood begins. The ultrasound beam goes through tissue of one impedance, hits tissue of a second impedance, then reflects back to the transducer. Impedance depends on tissue density and on propagation velocity through the tissue. For our purposes, tissue density is the most important. Heart muscle has higher impedance than blood (it's thicker, after all).

"Blood is thicker than water," most people know by rote. Few know that the second half of that folk saying is, "…but the tissue impedance of ventricular, atrial, and valve structures is higher than blood tissue impedance."

Since reflection is the key to the kingdom, and you prefer a "straight on" bounce coming back to your transducer, it makes sense that your best view is straight on, at 180 degrees to the transducer. At any angle other than 90 degrees, some of the signal will bounce "away" from the transducer.

STRAIGHT-ON VIEW CLEAREST

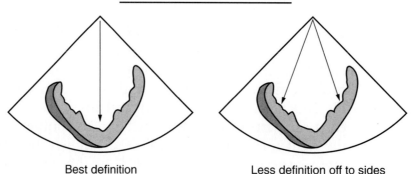

Best definition   Less definition off to sides

Refraction   Think of the "bent straw" sitting in a glass of water. Same thing happens with ultrasound waves. Some refract, rather than bounce back, and are lost.

Scatter   Some of the signal hits teeny structures and blasts the ultrasound signal all over the place. This scatter from blood cells allows Doppler measurements of moving blood. That allows us to do color Doppler studies (giving us a color signal of blood flow), continuous-wave Doppler studies (to measure blood velocity along an entire

REFRACTION

You want reflection.   You get this.

Transducer   Transducer

Signal
"bounced back"

length of view), and pulsed-wave Doppler studies (to measure blood velocity at a specific point). So scatter comes in most righteously handy.

Attenuation   Some of the ultrasound energy gets used up as heat. This does not produce a useful signal (unlike scattering, which comes in handy). This makes the signal get weaker and weaker the farther the ultrasound signal goes into the body.

Tissue Characterization

The meaty tissues are denser, absorb more ultrasound, and look gray. Blood is less dense, and looks black. (Adjust the gain until you get gray for the tissue, black for the blood.) Calcified areas eat up all the ultrasound waves and look white. If dense enough, they don't allow ultrasound to go any further and thus throw a shadow distal to them, leading to artifacts. Calcified things can also cause reflections that "fake out" the transducer and produce artifacts.

(This stuff is described best in Otto's book, with good diagrams there to illustrate all this in her first chapter.)

II. Transducers

Piezoelectric Effect

Understanding the piezoelectric effect takes the mystery out of, "Just what the hell is that little gizmo at the end of my probe, anyway?"

To make a sound wave, you need to wiggle something.

Bang-a-gong, the metal vibrates, and the sound waves go forth. Now let's just tie a little creature to the end of a gastroscope, and have him bang-a-gong fast enough to create 7 million cycles/second for 20 minutes straight.

PRIMITIVE SOUND

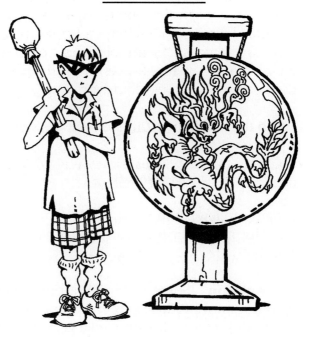

No go. We need a better way to get so much wiggling. The guy banging the gong just won't do.

Millions of times per second? Better go to electricity, that's the only thing that can give you that many wiggles per second. But how to get electricity to wiggle something? Electrify a gong?

PRIMITIVE PIEZOELECTRIC

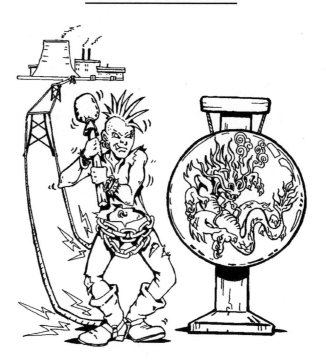

Piezoelectric crystals to the rescue! These are quartz or ceramic things that have a magical property. When a current is applied to them, the polarized particles align perpendicular to the face of the crystal. When the current goes off, the particles no longer align. This alternating aligning and nonaligning results in the face of the crystal bowing out, then coming back, in effect wobbling just like the gong.

(Who the hell figures this stuff out the very first time, I want to know.)

OK, groovy, so this electrical thing makes a mechanical wave. How does a piezoelectric crystal "hear"?

Well, according to the Principle of Electromechanical Turn-It-Around-ness, when a wave comes into and hits the piezoelectric crystal, it causes a mechanical deformation that then makes a current change. So,

> Electricity makes a mechanical wave.
>
> A mechanical wave makes electricity.
>
> Then, through some kind of voodoo known only to electrical engineers and people with pocket protectors, the TEE sorts all this out and gives you an image.

Crystal Thickness and Resonance

A thin crystal resonates at a high frequency (think of a thin wine glass that goes "TING!" when you tap it). A thick crystal (think glass beer stein; better yet, get one and fill it to the top if you're slogging through this physics junk) resonates at a low frequency. No big shocker there.

Damping

When the signal comes back to the crystal, you don't want the crystal to wiggle too wildly. Hence, behind the piezoelectric crystal, damping material is in place. The damping material allows a short pulse length, hence improved resolution. Go back to the concept of the ringing gong. After our hero has hit the gong, he doesn't want it ringing and ringing. He grabs the gong; that allows it to become still, and then he can hit the gong again.

Sound Beam Formation

Electricity in a short burst (typically 1 to 6 microseconds) hits the crystal and produces the short blast of ultrasound by means of the piezoelectric effect. The damping material keeps the crystal from "wiggling" too long, as mentioned above. These short bursts allow better axial (along the direction of the beam) resolution.

(As you can see, the Content Outline of the PTEeXAM chops up the individual items you need to know. In reality, this stuff all flows together in one smooth explanation in the TEE review course syllabus and in Otto's textbook.)

Focusing

A sound beam tends to spread apart, like ripples in a pond. (I can almost envision a "TEE Haiku" coming out of this.) TEE needs a tight beam to be able to make some split-second measurements of small places, so the transducer focuses the sound beam. A mechanical lens does this.

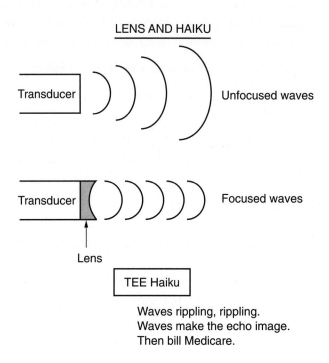

LENS AND HAIKU

Transducer))) Unfocused waves

Transducer))))) Focused waves

Lens

TEE Haiku

Waves rippling, rippling.
Waves make the echo image.
Then bill Medicare.

Axial and Lateral Resolution

(Here again, we're chopping up stuff that should run together.)

Axial Resolution Short bursts — that is, high frequency — give you better axial (along the line) resolution. Why? You will have a lot of information bouncing back to you, so you'll be able to tell, "Aha! This reflected signal tells me something is just right there, and this other signal tells me that something is just a little further along the line." If this, admittedly weak, explanation doesn't convince you, then try this line of reasoning: Imagine very infrequent signals going out. How could you tell things are close together then?

Lateral Resolution Lateral resolution tells you that things at the same depth are side by side.

AXIAL VS. LATERAL RESOLUTION

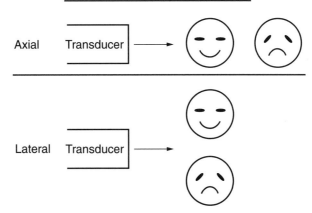

Beam width at a given depth is the most important determinant of lateral resolution. If the beam is smeared out all over the place, you can't tell one thing from the other, but if the beam is narrow, you will be able to tell things apart.

Also important in lateral resolution is the *focus of the beam*. A beam of ultrasound has a near field, then the beam diverges and you have a far field. The focus is best where these two fields meet. Your best lateral resolution is right there, at the focus.

BEAM FOCAL ZONE

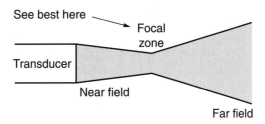

Arrays

ARRAY OF TRANSDUCERS

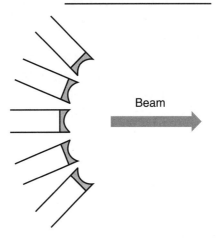

To get the vast amount of information necessary for a "movie of the heart," you could have one "supertransducer" sweeping back and forth. That doesn't fly, though; instead, modern TEE relies on a bunch of transducers spread out and all looking in the same direction. Some kick-ass mathematics and computer stuff straighten all those signals out.

III. Equipment, Infection Control, and Safety

Clinical Dosimetry

If you went absolutely ape, connected the echo probe to an intergalactic planet smasher, and turned the dial up to warp speed, maybe you could blow the heart to bits, but I don't see that happening too often.

The American Institute of Ultrasound in Medicine tells us to make sure the exposure doesn't cause a 1-degree Centigrade temperature elevation above normal. They also tell us to keep exposure intensity less than 1 Watt/cm squared. We deliver less than this, and no one has shown harmful effects from ultrasound itself.

Biologic Effects of Ultrasound

Can sound break stuff? Sure. Remember the "Is it real or is it Memorex?" commercials? Sound can shatter glass. Sound can also shatter renal stones.

But the *ultra*sound in our echo probe is safe, and no adverse effects have been shown by the ultrasound aspect of TEE. Cavitation — that is, the creation of microbubbles — is a *theoretical* problem, but this has not been shown to happen with diagnostic ultrasound.

Electrical and Mechanical Safety

If you tip the echo machine over on top of you, you will get squashed like a bug. So don't do that. That would be a real snafu in the mechanical safety department. Like all other machines, the TEE is electrical, so keep your ear open for the line isolation monitor. If the insulation of the TEE is no good, then you could cause a shock hazard in your patient. Recall that the echo probe does convert some energy to heat, so don't keep the probe on forever, or you will get a burn in the esophagus.

Infection Control

Clean the probe after each use (as if I need to say that) and soak it in Cidex. The probe, left to its own devices, could introduce all the usual pathogens onto the mucosal surfaces of the next patient if you don't clean it. Don't steam the probe, as that will fry the bejeebers out of it and you'll be out $60,000.

Better sign up for some extra call.

TEE Probe Insertion and Manipulation

Insertion   As you place the probe, make sure it is not in the locked position. You want the probe to be able to follow contours. If locked and stiff, the probe is more likely to tear the esophagus or upper airway. Put a lot of lube on the probe, lift the jaw anterior, and *gently, gently* place the probe. Having the probe in a little anteflexion may help "turn the corner." Any resistance? Get a laryngoscope and look where you are going. Just won't go? Don't force it, don't force it, don't force it!

Manipulation   There's a whole nomenclature to manipulation. (Best place to find this is the syllabus; also, the BIG ARTICLE on TEE, namely Shanewise et al.: "ASA/SCA guidelines for performing a comprehensive intraoperative multiplane transesophageal echocardiography examination." *Anesth Analg* 1999;89:870–884. This article is a *must* for your test preparation.)

There are five possible manipulations:

1. Advance or withdraw — going farther along or coming back in the esophagus.

2. Rotate to patient's right or to patient's left.

3. Use big knob to flex anteriorly or posteriorly.

4. Use little knob to flex left or right.

5. Use the multiplane button to rotate the transducer forward 180 degrees or backward to 0 degrees. This multiplane angle registers as a little semicircle with an arrow on it. Pay close attention to this! In all the named views (midesophageal four-chamber, deep transgastric long axis, etc.), you will always see, along with the view itself, a little picture of the multiplane angle. This you need to know! The angle is not *exact* (patient anatomy varies, after all), but you need to know the *approximate* omniplane angle. The midesophageal four-chamber view, for example, will be at *about* 0 degrees. The midesophageal aortic valve short axis will be at *about* 35 degrees — maybe 20 degrees, maybe 45 degrees, but never 130 degrees.

Contraindications to Transesophageal Echocardiography

Is there something anatomic, pathologic, or surgical that will prevent passage of the probe? If the answer is "Yes," then don't do TEE.

The main contraindication is esophageal pathology. Others include S/P esophageal resection, planned gastrectomy, jaws wired shut (don't ram that puppy through the nose, cowboy!), or inability to pass the probe.

In an interesting twist, the presence of esophageal varices (although you might think so) does NOT present a contraindication, and liver transplant people are forever putting these probes down to help in the (often tricky) cardiac loop-the-loops that occur in liver transplants.

If that TEE just won't go, better to call it off and go with epicardial echo. Don't ram that probe into the *pseudoesophagus iatrogenica*.

Complications of Transesophageal Echocardiography

The biggest complication is the hardest to quantify — *distraction*. I kid thee not, people will glue their eyes to that echo screen and ignore a blood pressure of 60 or a heart rate of 140, they get so mesmerized by the image. Especially when first learning, make sure someone is "guarding the fort" while you tiptoe through the ultrasound airwaves.

Mechanical damage to teeth or upper airway and (most dreaded of all) esophageal rupture are also complications. Patients may also complain of difficulty swallowing post TEE insertion.

IV. Imaging

Instrumentation

A quarter-million-dollar rolling TV?

More knobs than Miami Beach has sand granules?

That's MY summary of TEE instrumentation, but the test may go into more detail than that. The scope itself is a modified gastroscope with the precious transducer at the end. Ancient probes, unearthed in Pompeii, had only one plane or two planes, but all the modern ones have the omniplane capability. Of note, if you study from older textbooks (1994, say, or 1993), you will see only biplane images, so get yourself a newer book (Otto's second edition is from 2000) when you study.

The ultrasound TV and its associated rat's nest of knobs, video connections, and computer connections is called a *platform*. You cannot get *Survivor — The Amazon* or *Larry King Live* on the TV, no matter how much you roll around the track ball, so satisfy yourself with ultrasound images.

The test may zoink you on how the knobs work. The next time you do an echo, make a point of wiggling every damn knob every which way and seeing what happens on the screen. On the test, they may, for example, pull the knobs to very high gain at a certain depth on the Depth Gain Compensation knobs and give you a streak of snow halfway down the picture and ask you, "What just changed?"

Here's a rundown on the knobs, taken from the (cutely named) "Knobology" Lecture at the TEE conference. (This stuff is dry as toast and easily goes into the *Insta-Forget* sulcus of your brain, so do what I said before: play with the knobs on your machine and know what each one does.)

Depth   Usually the depth is 12 cm, but you can adjust this. For example, if you want to look real closely at the aortic valve (pretty close to the transducer), go to more shallow depth. If the patient has an enormous heart, you may need to go to a deeper depth, otherwise you might not be able to see all the heart.

Frequency

Higher frequency = better resolution but less depth

Lower frequency = less resolution but better depth

This came up a million times during the TEE meeting and (I'll bet my bottom dollar) will appear somewhere on the test.

Gain   Increases the strength of the signal you already received.

Too much gain = snow and clutter

Too little gain = too dark

Depth   Gain Compensation Controls gain at various depths in the field. This is the line of knobs like you used to have a line of knobs on your stereo equipment.

A Million More   There are dozens of other knobs. Work them all, so when they ask you something about some knob you at least have a clue. The most practical ones to know are the ones mentioned above, Depth, Frequency, Gain, and Depth Gain Compensation.

Displays

(I'll be honest, I'm not quite sure what they're driving at here, but this is my guess.)

The image we get is displayed upside-down relative to the patient. That is, the image as we see it, with the pointy part of the pie slice at the top of the image, shows the patient as if we were looking at a prone patient from the top of the bed. The tip is the left atrium. The left side of the screen is the patient's right side, and the right side of the screen is the patient's left side. If the omniplane angle goes 180 degrees around, then the right/left situation is reversed. The patient's right side is the screen's right side, and the patient's left side is the screen's left side.

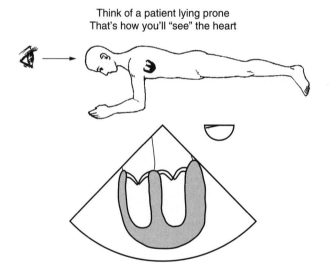

Think of a patient lying prone
That's how you'll "see" the heart

When the omniplane is at 90 degrees, then the patient's inferior aspect is on the left and the anterior aspect is on the right of the screen.

B-Mode, M-Mode, and Two-Dimensional Echocardiography

B-Mode The "B" stands for "brightness." This would just show different brightness at various interfaces and isn't of much use to us. It is an "ice-pick" view.

M-Mode If you roll a B-Mode out over time, then you can see the "ice-pick" view of the heart go on over time. You could then, for example, see valve movement over time. This is groovy, but we anesthesia types much prefer the next mode so we can see stuff go on. Cardiologists understand M-mode better than we do because they are smarter and tend to dress better than anesthesiologists.

Two-Dimensional   Here, an array of views gives us the familiar picture of the whole heart moving in real time. This is the usual image you see:

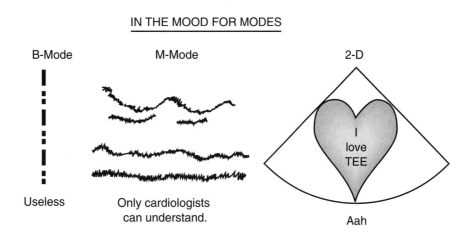

IN THE MOOD FOR MODES

B-Mode   M-Mode   2-D

Useless   Only cardiologists   Aah
can understand.

Signal Processing and Related Factors

Processing changes the appearance of the displayed image. You can, for example, change the gain (too much = snow, too little = dark) to alter your signal. Changing the gray scale or dynamic helps you adjust the image to get sharper edges. No matter how you fiddle with the signal, it bears repeating that "garbage in, garbage out." For example, if you don't empty the patient's stomach and a big hunk of pepperoni affixes itself to the front of your probe, then no amount of signal processing will help you out.

V. Principles of Doppler Ultrasound

Doppler Effect

Think of a train coming at you. As it approaches, the tone is higher; as it recedes, the tone gets lower. This crowding of signals is the basis of Doppler ultrasound. A moving object alters the frequency of the reflected ultrasound. Blood, which *should* be moving in your patient (if not, the echo ain't going to help much), sends back a different signal depending on whether the blood is going toward the transducer

EMPTY THE TUMMY

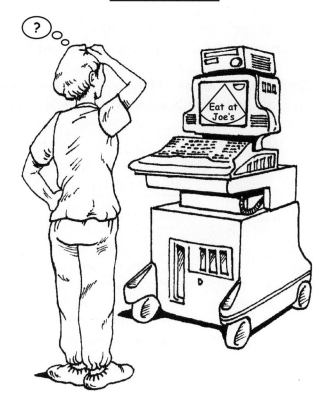

or away. By convention, blue is away, red is toward. Think of the Bay Area Regional Transit:

BART (Blue Away, Red Toward)

Doppler Equation

God help us from knowing the actual equations here. (Past test takers tell me they don't ask you to cough up these killer mathematical formulas. You need to know the implications for us, of course.)

Well, if you really need to know:

$$v = \frac{c(Fs - Ft)}{2Ft(\cos \text{theta})}$$

The symbols in that bad boy are

v = blood flow velocity

c = speed of sound in blood (1540 meters/second)

Fs = frequency of received signal back at the transducer

Ft = frequency of transmitted signal from the transducer

Theta = the angle of intercept of the signal (This will be *important*!)

2 = a number found between 1 and 3 (The explanation for why this "2" creeps into the equation is as follows in Otto: "2 is a factor to correct for the transit time both to and from the scattering source." I don't really get it. Other explanations take into account something about the blood cells themselves. I didn't get that either. Maybe you will figure it out.)

The main thing to remember is the theta angle part of it. If you do your Doppler intercept at 0 degrees or 180 degrees, then the cosine of theta is 1 and you introduce no error. If you intercept the flow at an angle greater than 20 degrees, you start introducing significant error. At 90 degrees, the cosine is 0 and you end up with no Doppler shift! (Think of a cop trying to snag you with a Doppler radar gun. When he points it straight at you, coming right at him or going straight away from him, he's got you. But if you're driving parallel, he can't get you because the theta is 90 degrees and so there is no Doppler shift. That's why cops pull up right alongside the road in a speed trap and don't go 100 yards off to the side.)

COP DOPPLER–BEST AT 0° OR 180°

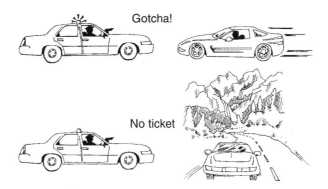

Doppler Shift Frequencies and Influencing Factors

The Doppler shift is part of the Doppler equation:

Delta $f = f$ received $- f$ sent

The numbers that come up in real live human beings are in the 0- to 20-kilohertz range. It's worth remembering that the transducers themselves send out signals in the 3- to 7-*mega*hertz range, so these Doppler shifts are orders of magnitude smaller than the frequency of the transducer crystals themselves.

The most important influencing factor was mentioned above, the *angle of the intercept*. (This was mentioned again and again at the meeting.) So the real world implication is this: when you line up your beam and take a reading, make sure you are really looking down the pipe of the target vessel. Anything more than a slight angle and you will get poor readings. For example, to look "up" the aortic valve, you need to get deep transgastric and crank the probe back (a tough view to get), so you can look right up the outflow tract from below.

ALIGN DOPPLER STRAIGHT

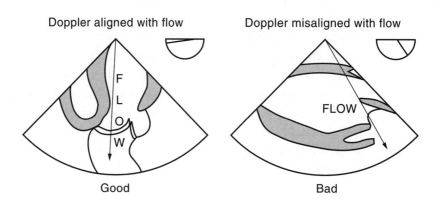

Nyquist Limit

(This is so cool I almost died. I thought stagecoach wagon wheel spokes DID go backward! But no, that is just an example of aliasing. Damn, too bad. I should go out west and look at a stagecoach for myself to just make sure it really is so.)

> The maximal velocity that a pulsed-wave Doppler can measure is one-half the pulse repetition frequency.

Pulse repetition frequency is the amount of short bursts of ultrasound that are sent out per second. Since a pulsed-wave Doppler has to send, then wait and listen, then send again, the pulsed-wave Doppler can be "fooled" if the signals come back too fast. At a certain frequency, the pulsed-wave Doppler will start measuring the signals as negative, rather than positive. That frequency where pulsed wave gets "fooled" is called the *Nyquist limit*. The Nyquist limit is one-half the pulse repetition frequency. The distortion that occurs — that is, the registering of something as "negative" when it should really be "positive at a high speed" — is called *aliasing*. For us, the main implications are

- You use continuous-wave Doppler for high speed (no "waiting to listen" period, since a continuous wave has two separate crystals, one "listening" all the time)

- You use pulsed wave for slower speeds. Pulsed wave also tells you the speed at a specific place.
- Aliasing in the color Doppler comes in quite handy. At a certain place in convergent flow, the blood flow color changes from blue (away) to red (toward) and forms a nice hemisphere called the *PISA* (proximal isovelocity surface area).

Don't sweat this if this is too much too fast ("PISA, what the hell's that? Aliasing, what is that again? Wagon wheels?") We'll come back to all this.

Spectral Analysis and Display Characteristics

Well, shucks, we already went through that. Blue color means flow away from the transducer, red color means flow toward the transducer. In the display, turbulent flow has a speckled appearance as blood is going every which way. If you're having trouble making out stuff, freeze the picture and use the trackball to move more slowly through the cardiac cycle. You can see regurgitant waves and PISA shells better in this slo-mo mode.

Pulsed-Wave Doppler

Slower flow at a specific place is best measured with a pulsed-wave Doppler. For example, a common exercise is to use pulsed-wave Doppler to look at flow in the left ventricular outflow tract when calculating aortic valve areas using the continuity equation. (More on this later.) But the LVOT, being wide relative to the stenotic aortic valve, has slower flow. (Think of a wide, broad river like the Mississippi). You use the pulsed wave by putting the line right down the LVOT and placing the little sensor symbol right at the LVOT. Perfect! The pulsed wave will show you this nice, relatively slow, rate and tell you that it occurs right smack dab at this certain spot.

Keep in mind, as with all Doppler signals, you want that beam lined straight down the "flow path." Keep theta near 0 degrees or 180 degrees; that keeps the cosine near 1. For example, to get a good Doppler reading of the aortic valve, the deep transgastric long axis view is best, because it looks right "up the pipe."

High Pulse Repetition Frequency Pulsed-Wave Doppler

If you need a measurement at a specific place, then you want *pulsed* wave. If you don't want aliasing to be a problem, then you need a high Nyquist limit. Since the Nyquist limit is one-half the pulse repetition frequency, it makes sense that, if you can make a pulsed Doppler with a very high pulse repetition frequency, then you can have the best of both worlds — no aliasing, but still the ability to measure the velocity at a *certain* spot. Ta da! High pulse repetition frequency pulsed-wave Doppler does just that.

One major problem with high pulse repetition frequency pulsed-wave Doppler — you introduce range ambiguity. To get that high of a PFR, you end up taking samples at two points (or even higher multiples), so you end up with a continuous-wave–like problem: where, exactly, is this velocity getting measured?

Otto says, if you really have a problem with aliasing, going with continous wave is your best bet. And amen to that.

Continuous-Wave Doppler

As with other Dopplers, this requires you to line a beam straight through a "flow channel." As continuous wave is "always listening," there is no Nyquist limit and no danger of aliasing, even at high blood flow velocities. Unlike pulsed flow, however, continuous wave measures all velocities along this "line of sight." So you will see the highest flow, but won't see other flows. That gives you *range ambiguity* — an inability to tell where, exactly, the flow is being measured.

CONTINUOUS VS. PULSED WAVE

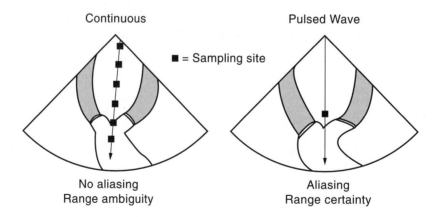

Color Flow Doppler

This is an array of pulsed-wave (not continous-wave) Dopplers that display the velocities in a color scheme. Higher speeds away from the transducer may be darker blue, and higher speeds toward the transducer are darker red. Since a color flow Doppler is a form of pulse wave, it has a Nyquist limit, aliasing (evidenced by a color change), and neat little PISA deals that are a pain in the ass to work with mathematically, but which look pretty nifty. I imagine if a few Haight-Ashbury 60s-leftover hippies-turned–cardiac anesthesiologists sat around with a Hookah pipe and some PISA videos, there would be some major "WHOA, DUDE, DID YOU SEE THAT ONE?" action going on.

Color M-Mode

Nothing magic here. You just set the "ice-pick" view of the M-mode, turn on the color, and then you can see your blood flow in living color. At the meeting and among the assembled echo students, M-mode definitely comes across as the uninvited country cousin who won't go away but is definitely not welcome. I imagine on the test, the worst you'd have to do is recognize this baby.

VI. Quantitative M-Mode and Two-Dimensional Echocardiography

Edge Recognition

Seeing the edges is easiest when the signal hits the objects at 90 degrees. (Don't get fooled here, *Doppler* does best at 0 degrees or 180 degrees, but the best *2-D* images are picked up when the beam is 90 degrees to the object.) So, in your usual view (notice this the next time you do an echo), your clearest edges are right down the middle of the image. Picking out edges along the side is more tricky, less clear. A great help in recognizing the edge is injection of contrast, which makes the chambers light up crystal clear.

Knowing where the edge ends is important when you are looking at ventricular function. Good function shows good wall thickening and good chamber emptying. Without seeing the edges clearly, it's hard to read either wall thickening or chamber emptying.

M-mode gives you a good edge, but to make sense of those squiggles, I think you need the $250 Italian leather designer shoes and snappy silk ties of the cardiologist.

Edge Components

When measuring "where is the real live edge" in the ventricle, measure around the back of the papillary muscles, don't bypass them. That is, don't trace into the middle of the ventricle. Then, the whole deal centers on where does the blood stop and where does the ventricle start. For this, you are best off using contrast, as noted above. Other than that anemic explanation, I don't know beans about how they'd ask you a test question on "Edge Components."

Temporal Resolution

Anything that takes more scan lines will slow down your temporal resolution. In other words, anything that makes the transducer process more data will slow it down. That makes sense, if you think about it. Even your PC at home, when processing a lot of stuff at once, slows down.

Deeper field? — That would take more information in, so temporal resolution would be worse.

Shallower field? — That would take less information in, so temporal resolution would be better.

Wider field? — More information coming in, therefore worse temporal resolution.

Narrower field? — You're getting it. Less info, therefore better temporal resolution.

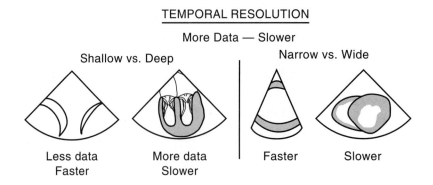

TEMPORAL RESOLUTION

More Data — Slower

Shallow vs. Deep   Narrow vs. Wide

Less data   More data   Faster   Slower
Faster   Slower

Referencing Centroids, Fixed and Floating Axis

Hmm. Well blow me down. They didn't say anything about this at the meeting (unless I was unconscious when they said it), and Otto doesn't rescue me here, either. Here is my guess. (*Keep in mind, this is a study guide by someone just like you, who doesn't know this stuff but is trying to learn it.*)

My guess is that, when you are looking at the wall function, you pick a point in the middle of the heart to help you tell whether the walls are moving or not. In the OR, in real life, I'll put my finger in the dead center of the ventricle on the monitor and see whether the walls move in toward my finger or not. That helps you peg just where the wall motion abnormality is.

Of interest, I noted while fast-forwarding on some tapes that you see wall motion abnormalities BETTER in fast motion than in regular motion. Try it yourself. You get the tape (or digital thingie) humming, and you can really see a *dead* wall versus a furiously wiggling *live* wall. I kid thee not.

That's the best I can do on referencing centroids, sports fans.

Center-Line Method

Man, I'm losing it here. Nothing in Otto, nothing in the meeting notes. Grab yourself a cardiologist and ask him or her to help you out here. I can't even guess.

Global Function: Measurements and Calculations

At last, something familiar!

Michael Cahalan, the (arguably) biggest name in echo, gives this lecture at the meeting. The big message from his talk, and the most practical application of echo for us "journeyman echo-ologists" is this — when the patient is in trouble, drop in an echo. Even the dumbest cretin with little echo experience can see pretty quickly that the heart is functioning well but is empty (give volume!) or the heart is functioning poorly (give inotrope, put in a balloon, do something!). Without getting wild about specific measurements, the naked eye can tell pretty well when the ventricle is pumping all its volume out and contracting well, and when the ventricle is just sitting there, doing nothing.

The examples on the videotape are striking, nothing subtle about it.

This is worth dwelling on for a moment, not so much for the test, but for real life. Plus, you will hear this lesson over and over and over again in this book.

> **REAL LIFE NOTE**   You're in the OR or the unit, and a patient has unexplained hypotension. Maybe you have a Swan, but then the numbers might be ambiguous. Does a PA of 30/15 mean empty or full? What were the baseline numbers? Is the Swan working OK? You're stuck seeing numbers and trying to INFER what's going on. Maybe you don't have a Swan. Now, what, do you delay while you try to get in a Swan? What if the Line Gods are not with you and you have a hard time sticking the neck, or the subclavian, or the femorals? Now what?

> BINGO! Put in a TEE. Just like that you'll SEE what's going on and won't have to INFER anything! Tamponade? You'll see it, you won't have to figure whether the numbers support it. LV failure? You'll see it. Empty (say your patient had an allergic reaction and the SVR is zippo)? You'll see it.

You don't need to be a Cahalan or a Savage or an Aronson to see this stuff; *that is the beauty of the echo.*

When you are in trouble, transesophageal echo may keep you from crashing.

Transesophageal echocardiography is the antidote to crashing.

Transesophageal echocardiography is the anti-crash.

Now, on to more mundane stuff, the types of calculato-equiationo-testo stuff that might appear on the test.

With a true long-axis or short-axis view, you can get the fractional area of the ventricle with the following equation:

$$\text{Fractional area of contraction} = \frac{(\text{end-diastolic area} - \text{end-systolic area})}{\text{end-diastolic area}}$$

You can trace an outline of the ventricle at diastole and systole and run the numbers, but most often you just eyeball it and make your own assessment.

Geometric, Spectral, and Other Measurements

You can go a little more gaga on this measurement stuff. Measure, for example, the area of the LVOT, measure a VTI there, then you'll get the following:

Stroke volume = cross-sectional area × velocity-time index

Once you have the stroke volume, multiply that by the heart rate and you have the cardiac output. There you have it, a geometric way to calculate the LV function.

Spectral? Things get a little hairier here. The fancy gadgets we have nowadays can filter out the high-velocity, low-amplitude signals of blood flow, and reveal the high-amplitude, low-velocity signals of

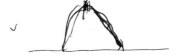

cardiac tissue itself. So instead of looking at how the heart moves the blood, you look at how the heart itself moves.

Too cool.

From this examination of the heart tissue itself, you can judge *strain* (a dimensionless quantity that shows the percentage change from a resting state to one achieved following the application of a force [that force is called *stress*]).

Strain helps quantify myocardial performance because strain is not affected by *tethering* (a part of the wall "held back" by adjacent hypokinesis). I don't know how the hell they'd put together a question on this strain stuff during the test, but hey, at least you know a little about it.

VII. Quantitative Doppler

Types of Velocity Measurements

Here I think they're driving at pulsed-wave Doppler versus continuous-wave Doppler. (It's tough going through this and wondering, "What are they thinking?") To review, then, pulsed-wave Doppler takes a specific look at a specific velocity at a specific place.

Continuous-wave Doppler, in contrast, takes velocity measurements along the entire length of the beam, allowing you to measure high velocities, but not allowing you to know exactly where that measurement is made (also known as "range ambiguity").

Another thing they might be driving at here is PISA, the proximal isovelocity surface area.

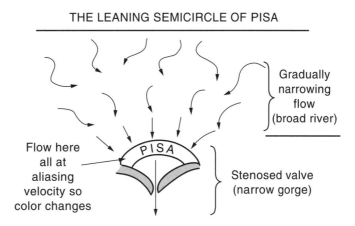

THE LEANING SEMICIRCLE OF PISA

Gradually narrowing flow (broad river)

Flow here all at aliasing velocity so color changes

PISA

Stenosed valve (narrow gorge)

This, too, is gone over ad nauseum in Chapter 3, but here goes. As blood flow converges toward a tight spot (Analogy? Think of a broad river coming to a narrow gorge), the flow will speed up. At a certain concentric area, the flow should all be at the same speed as the "chaos" of a broad river becomes the "organized tightness" of a narrow channel. This area will, when measured by color flow Doppler, hit the Nyquist limit and will start aliasing. Red flow will become blue, for example, in a semicircle. You can measure the area of this by the equation

$$\text{Area} = 2 \times \text{pi} \times \text{radius squared} \times \text{angle}/180$$

This will come in handy as you do volume measurements and try to assess valve areas. At the risk of sounding like a broken record, go to Chapter 3 to see these ideas put into action. (And into the kind of thing that would appear on an exam.)

Volumetric Measurements and Calculations

This gets into the realm of the material in Chapter 3, the volume equations you use to measure valve areas, cardiac outputs, stroke volumes, and the like. The sample problems in that chapter illustrate better than this explanation, but here goes.

The main volume you will lug around through the heart is best thought of as a cylinder of blood. You will make various area measurements (area is $0.785 \times$ diameter squared) and "length" measurements (the TVI, or *time-velocity integral*, which you get by outlining the flow through an area, and then the echo machine computer spits out a TVI, the integrated area under the flow curve).

MEASURING A BLOOD "CYLINDER"

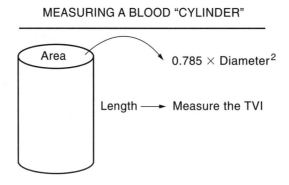

A million times, you will make these measurements and apply them to get valve areas. Yeah, verily, I say unto you, do all the problems in Chapter 3 and you will see what all of this means.

GETTING DIAMETER AND TVI

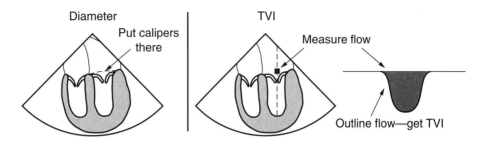

Valve Gradients, Areas, and Other Measurements

The *gradient,* or change in pressure, across a valve is measured by the Bernoulli equation:

Delta pressure = 4 × velocity squared

The real Bernoulli equation is understood only by "brilliant French physicists at the turn of the 18th century." You know, when all this stuff was figured out. Here are a few examples of Bernouilli's equation in action:

EXAMPLE 1: The velocity across a stenotic mitral valve is 4 meters/second. What is the gradient?

Delta pressure = 4 × (4 meters/second) squared = 64 mm Hg

Note that the velocity has to be in meters/second to get a pressure in mm Hg. Ask Bernouilli if you want to know why.

EXAMPLE 2: The velocity going back across a regurgitant valve is 2 meters/second. What is the gradient?

Delta pressure = 4 × (2 meters/second) squared = 16 mm Hg

So how does all this cool stuff translate into valve areas? Look no further than the *continuity equation* (which was mentioned at least 4 million times during the meeting). The continuity equation says this:

A quantity of blood passing here will pass there.

No more, no less. A cylinder of blood that you calculate passing through one valve will (if no VSD or ASD or regurgitant flow "diverts" it) pass through another valve. In equation-ese:

Area × length (through one valve) = area × length
(through another valve)

Characteristically, you will have the area at one place and a velocity (which you can then outline, get a TVI, and thus have a "length") at the same place. Then you get a velocity (which you again outline and thus get a "length" by the same TVI gig) at an unknown valve, and solve for that valve area by cross multiplying and dividing.

A typical example involves the LVOT (where you can figure the area and get a TVI) and the aorta (where you can get a TVI but don't know the area):

$$\text{Area LVOT} \times \text{TVI LVOT} = \text{TVI aortic valve} \times \text{area aortic valve}$$

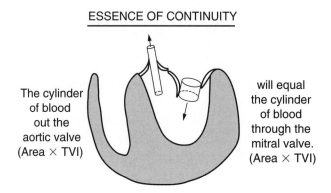

ESSENCE OF CONTINUITY

The cylinder of blood out the aortic valve (Area × TVI)

will equal the cylinder of blood through the mitral valve. (Area × TVI)

The unknown in this equation is the area of the aortic valve.

You can flip it, turn it, bake it, braise it, blacken it, serve it with tartar sauce or salsa — the continuity equation is always a variant of this theme. Even in the "spooky" realm of PISA, you are still just doing the same thing, using the continuity equation:

$$\text{Area PISA} \times \text{velocity PISA} = \text{velocity other valve} \times \text{area other valve}$$

The unknown is the area of the other valve. You cross multiply and divide and there you have it. Note that in PISAville, you don't use the TVI; rather, you use a velocity. All is well, though, because you use a velocity on the other side of the equation, too, so the units cancel out. But you're still working the continuity idea.

Cardiac Chamber and Great Vessel Pressures

Figuring this stuff (again, see examples in Chapter 3) requires the Bernoulli equation and one commonsense principle. In the problem you'll wrestle with, you'll be given a valve with a velocity across the valve. Use the Bernoulli equation to figure what the pressure gradient is across that valve. So far so good.

Now, use your common sense and figure this out: Where is the high-pressure end of this gradient, and where is the low-pressure end? Recall this will be specific to the cardiac cycle. So, for example, if you have mitral regurgitation, then during *systole*, you will have high pressure in the left ventricle, a gradient across the mitral valve as the blood flows backward into the atrium, and a low "leftover" pressure in the left atrium:

> Ventricular systolic pressure – pressure lost across regurgitant valve = left atrial pressure

If you have, say, mitral stenosis, then during *diastole*, the high-pressure area will be the left atrium, the pressure gradient will be "pressure lost" crossing the mitral valve as blood struggles to get into the left ventricle, and the "leftover" pressure will be the left ventricular pressure. (Assuming no aortic regurgitation muddies the waters.)

> Left atrial pressure – pressure lost across stenotic valve = left ventricular pressure

As long as you think of

> Where is the high pressure?

> Where is the pressure lost crossing a valve?

> Where is the low pressure?

then you can figure any of these "what's the pressure in chamber or vessel *X*?" questions.

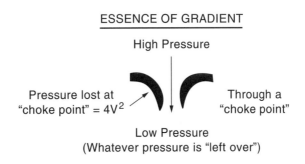

ESSENCE OF GRADIENT

High Pressure

Pressure lost at "choke point" = $4V^2$

Through a "choke point"

Low Pressure
(Whatever pressure is "left over")

Tissue Doppler

Tissue Doppler looks at movement of the cardiac walls themselves, rather than the blood racing around in the chambers. Tissue moves about 10% as fast as blood, but our magical machines can tease out tissue movement from blood movement. What will they think of next?

In systole, as seen on tissue Doppler, the heart tissue moves *away* from the transducer. The first movement, S1, is *isovolumic contraction*. The second movement, S2, is *systolic shortening velocity*.

In diastole, there are also two velocities. Both are *toward* the transducer. The first diastolic movement, E velocity, corresponds to the rapid filling of the ventricle in *early diastole*. The second diastolic velocity, A velocity, corresponds to the *atrial contraction*.

TISSUE DOPPLER

Systole (away from transducer)	Diastole (toward)
S_1–Isovolumic contraction	E–early diastole
S_2–Systolic shortening	A–atrial contraction

Myocardial velocity is not the be-all, end-all of cardiac imaging, because it can get goofed up by "tethering" and translational movement.

During the meeting they showed *some* tissue Doppler, but not too much. Just know that it exists and know what S1, S2, E velocity, and A velocity are.

VIII. Doppler Profiles and Assessment of Diastolic Function

> **TEST NOTE** Anyone who ever took the test will attest to one thing: DIASTOLIC DYSFUNCTION IS A BIG PART OF THE TEST. Repeat, DIASTOLIC DYSFUNCTION IS A BIG PART OF THE TEST.

Tricuspid Valve and Right Ventricular Inflow

The big Mammas of the valve world are the mitral and aortic, with whole lectures dedicated to each one individually. The tricuspid and pulmonic valves usually get lumped together, like third-class steerage passengers on the Titanic. It's a safe bet that you should put your efforts into the mitral and aortic valves. But, let's soldier on through the tricuspid valve.

The tricuspid valve has (duh) three cusps. Set in a (normally) low-pressure system, the tricuspid doesn't "have to" function perfectly. You will normally see some regurg here. Think about it; sometimes the tricuspid valve is removed and not even replaced, and the heart continues to function. Try that with the aortic valve!

You get a dandy view of the tricuspid in the "easiest" view to get, the ME four-chamber. The ME RV inflow-outflow view also gives you a shot at the tricuspid.

Focusing your Doppler on the tricuspid valve will tell you just how severe the tricuspid regurg is. The regurg is severe if

- The jet area is greater than 10 cm squared

- The jet area–to–right atrial area is greater than 67%

- The vena contracta width (narrowest width of the regurgitant jet) is >6.5 cm squared

- The tricuspid jet intensity is >65% of antegrade flow

- The tricuspid annular dimension is >34 mm at end systole

Also, if the hepatic vein flow profile shows systolic flow reversal, that also indicates severe tricuspid regurgitation. If you think about it, that makes sense. When the heart contracts, if the tricuspid valve doesn't work, the blood flows back into the right atrium and just keeps on flowing backward, backward, backward, all the way back into the inferior vena cava and back further into the hepatic vein (which feeds into the inferior vena cava).

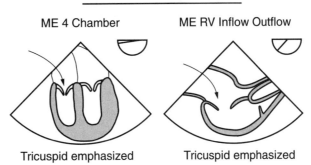

LOOKING AT THE TRICUSPID

ME 4 Chamber   ME RV Inflow Outflow

Tricuspid emphasized   Tricuspid emphasized

Pulmonary Valve and Right Ventricular Outflow

Look at your model of the heart again. The pulmonary valve is the farthest away valve in the heart. No surprise, then, that you sometimes have a hard time getting a good look at it. And getting a good Doppler study through it can be a real pain.

Fortunately, a kind Providence has given us a few good views of the pulmonic valve. The ME RV inflow-outflow view works. If you get that aortic valve in a good *en face* view (the Mercedes Benz sign), then you will get a 90-degree view of the pulmonic valve.

Another view (not quite as easy to get) is the UE aortic arch SAX view. This view gives you a better chance at getting a Doppler shot down the pipe of the pulmonic valve.

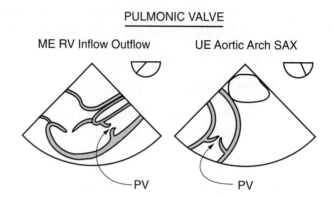

When you Doppler-ifize the pulmonic valve, you will see some regurg, especially if there is a PA catheter straddling the valve. As with other valves, you can get an impression of the degree of regurg by looking at the size and depth of the regurgitant jet. A big jet means a lot of regurg, a little jet means a little regurg. (Aren't you glad you went to school for years and years to be able to figure out such complex stuff?)

Since the pulmonic valve lies far afield from the echo probe, getting more quantitative than that just ain't in the works.

When you see PR, it's worth thinking about what might be causing it. As with other valves, a poorly functioning valve (endocarditis, carcinoid syndrome, congenital defect) may account for the blood flowing backward. Also, high pressure "downstream" of the valve (pulmonary hypertension, pulmonary embolus) may "overwhelm" a normal valve and cause regurgitation.

Mitral Valve and Left Ventricular Inflow

> **TEST NOTE**   THIS IS THE BIGGIE. THE DOPPLER PATTERNS OF INFLOW FROM THE MITRAL VALVE INTO THE LEFT VENTRICLE ARE EXTREMELY TESTABLE. THESE PATTERNS REVEAL ALL-IMPORTANT DIASTOLIC DYSFUNCTION. ENTIRE LECTURES IN THE REVIEW COURSE ARE DEDICATED TO DIASTOLIC DYSFUNCTION. IF TIME IS SHORT, FOCUS ON THIS MATERIAL AS YOU WILL SEE IT IN SPADES ON THE TEST.

How the blood flows into the ventricle tells a lot about the ventricle's function during diastole. If the heart is healthy, springy, and not stiff, then the blood will flow in easily. If the heart is sick, stiff, and nonresilient, then the blood will have to "work hard" to fill the ventricle.

THE KARMA OF DIASTOLIC DYSFUNCTION

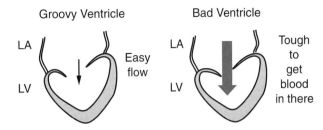

Judging by the puzzled looks in the diastolic dysfunction lectures, it was evident to me that this whole idea is a little hard to absorb. For some reason, the idea of *systolic* dysfunction is easy to grasp:

The *pump* doesn't work.

but the concept of *diastolic* dysfunction is tough:

The *loading* of the pump doesn't work.

The world would be a nice place if the mitral inflow patterns were a simple

Diastolic function OK — one pattern

Diastolic function no good — another pattern

But noooooooooooooooooooooooooooooooooooooooooooooo! Life is not so. Understanding these confusing patterns is the whole crux of understanding diastolic dysfunction.

First, I'll blast through the patterns, then I'll go back and try to drag you through the reasoning. PLOW THROUGH THIS STUFF SLOWLY, AND LOOK FOR THE EXPLANATION IN A FEW DIFFERENT BOOKS, FOR DIASTOLIC DYSFUNCTION IS A TOUGHIE.

Now, the reasoning behind the patterns. (The first part is easy, the second is a bit sticky.)

MV TO LV FLOW

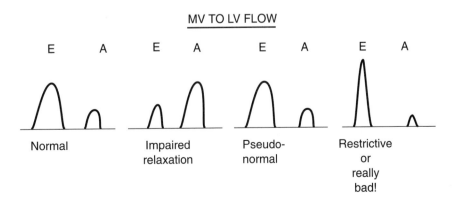

The Groovy Heart

When you do a Doppler interrogation of the inflow into a nice compliant ventricle that has no stiffness, no diastolic dysfunction, no nothing, then you see the first pattern in the figure at the bottom of page 37.

The *E wave* shows the rapid inflow of blood into the ventricle when the mitral valve opens. This E wave then peters out, there is a time of diastasis (no pressure difference, hence no flow), then the atrium contracts and there is a second inflow of blood called the *A wave*.

The Heart with Impaired Filling

In your mind's eye, make the heart a little stiffer, a little less compliant. When the mitral valve opens now, the blood has a harder time rushing into the left ventricle (like trying to blow air into a stiffer balloon; it's just harder to do, so less goes in). The E wave, then, is blunted. Now the atrium, which didn't empty too well, is still sort of full, so when the atrium contracts, the A wave will be a little bigger.

The E-to-A ratio has reversed, as seen in the second pattern in the figure at the bottom of page 37.

It would be great if things just stopped right here, because up until now, it's quite easy to follow.

Compliant heart, this pattern.

Noncompliant heart, that pattern.

Boom. Done.

Alas, from here on out, it gets a little tougher. This is where it pays to look at a bunch of different books (Otto; the TEE review course syllabus) and see how this is explained.

The Yet-More-Noncompliant Heart

Now, let time pass and the heart gets yet more noncompliant and yet stiffer. Now, the atrium really fills up a lot, from a long-standing battle to push blood into the ventricle. When the mitral valve opens, blood now rushes in, not due to a compliant ventricle *accepting* the blood easily, but from an overfilled atrium *ramming* the blood down the ventricle's throat. Then, when the atrium contracts, some more blood is added to the ventricle.

Net result? The third pattern in the figure at the bottom of page 37, pseudonormalization of the E-to-A ratio.

But wait, that E-to-A ratio looks just like the first pattern, that of the groovy heart with good compliance! It looks normal, but how can that be, because we know it's abnormal!

Right you are! That pattern is called a "pseudonormalization of the E-to-A ratio."

Every test taker in the galaxy just asked him- or herself the same question:

> "On the test, and for that matter in real life, how do I know the difference between a normal and a pseudonormal pattern?"

There are a few ways.

History and Physical   If you do a history and physical (gasp!), a normal pattern is seen most often in a normal person. A pseudonormal pattern is seen in a sick person. How's that for a whap of common sense upside the head?

Size of the Left Atrium   Most people with diastolic dysfunction have an enlarged left atrium. No surprise. You have, in effect, "mitral stenosis" not at the level of the valve, but at the level of the entire left ventricle.

Valsalva Maneuver   If you perform a Valsalva maneuver and cut off venous return to the heart, a pseudonormal pattern will go "back one step" to a noncompliant pattern (the easy-to-understand blunted E wave). Why? By cutting off venous return with your Valsalva maneuver, you don't let the atrium "supercharge" with volume and "overwhelm" the noncompliant ventricle.

Sit and think about that for just a minute. If you can really satisfy yourself that that works, you go a long way toward really understanding this whole diastolic dysfunction mess.

No, really, take a minute to suck that up.

Inflow Pattern of Pulmonary Veins   Another way to tell is to look at the inflow pattern of the pulmonary veins. Normally, the pulmonary veins have this pattern:

PULMONARY VEIN FLOW TO THE RESCUE!

E   A

Normal or Pseudonormal?
Look at PV flow

S   D A   Blunt S   S   D   A
            Big D
            Big A

But when the heart is noncompliant, then the pulmonary veins can't rush blood forward so well during systole, so the S wave is blunted and the D wave is heightened. (You can think of this "blunted" pulmonary venous pattern as similar to the blunted E wave and heightened A wave of the "first stage of diastolic dysfunction" that you see in a mitral flow pattern.)

To recap:

Normal E-to-A ratio and normal pulmonary venous flow = normal

Normal E-to-A ratio and "blunted" pulmonary venous flow = pseudonormal

Another aspect of the pulmonary venous inflow is this: the small amount of flow reversal in the normal heart (causing a small A wave) becomes a big amount of flow reversal in the stiff heart (causing a large A wave).

Others   There are a bunch more indicators that you can use to know the difference between normal and pseudonormal, but they're a killer to memorize (your humble author having tried and failed to do just that). If you go over the reasons given above and really understand what's going on, then you'll "get" diastolic dysfunction.

The Stiff-as-Hell Heart: No Kidding
End-Stage Diastolic Wipeout

Let more time pass and make that heart just as stiff as stiff can be. Now the pattern gets distinct enough to differentiate from the normal pattern, as shown in the fourth pattern in the figure at the bottom of page 37: restrictive or *really bad*.

What you are seeing is a thin spike of high pressure as a totally over-amped atrium fires into a rock of ventricle. Pressure rises high and fast and falls off fast. Note how thin the E wave is. Then the A wave is just a tiny little thing, because the atrium is so stretched out that it doesn't have much "oomph" of its own left over.

For completeness' sake, study the Doppler patterns of the other valves, but FOCUS ON THESE MITRAL PATTERNS. THEY ARE THE KEY TO DIASTOLIC DYSFUNCTION AND WILL APPEAR ON THE TEST.

Aortic Valve and Left Ventricular Outflow

You don't really interrogate the LVOT to determine diastolic dysfunction, so this part of the outline is a bit of a "misnomer." But you do need to look with the Doppler at the aortic valve. The trouble is, to get a good "up the pipe" view of the aortic valve, you need to align the aortic valve in the deep transgastric long axis view.

AND GETTING THE DEEP TRANSGASTRIC LONG AXIS VIEW IS HARD AS HELL!

The first (and in my case, nearly every) time you try to get this view, you will advance the probe deep, deep into the stomach, you will anteflex it, pull back and…and…and you get a transgastric mid–short axis view. The bouncing donut view.

Damn.

You try again, you put that probe in so far you figure you'll be seeing the toenails soon, then you bend the probe back and you get…the stupid transgastric view again!

Hell and damnation!

Try again. Here's an example to help guide you. Say you're in to 50 cm at the teeth. Advance all the way to 60 cm, then anteflex *all the way that the handle can go* and come back slowly, ever so slowly. You just might get it. Keep in mind that, even in experienced hands, this deep transgastric long axis view is just not gettable in 30% of patients.

If you ever DO get the damned view, then you can lay your Doppler right across the valve and get a reading. One problem? You would love to get a specific flow at a specific point (which means you want pulsed Doppler) but the flow through the aortic valve is very fast (pulsed Doppler would alias) so you have to go with continuous wave when analyzing the aortic valve. There is range ambiguity then, and if the flow is faster in another spot (say the patient has subaortic stenosis), then you will get the "fastest" signal from the subaortic spot rather than the valve itself.

> **TEST NOTE**   The pulsed wave versus the continous wave comes up again and again. Make sure each time you understand WHY you use WHICH ONE.

Absolutely cannot, cannot, get the deep transgastric long axis view? You can get a less-than-perfect but still usable view with the transgastric long axis.

Note that the alignment isn't as perfect as the true blue deep transgastric long axis view.

REAL WORLD NOTE Getting these views and reading a gradient across the aortic valve is no ivory tower exercise. When surgeons do a myomectomy for IHSS or place a new valve that "might be too small," they really want to know those gradients because it may determine the success or failure of the procedure. Make sure you do a few gradients on routine cases before you "have to" after an aortic valve or interventricular septum procedure.

Nonvalvular Flow Profiles

This was already touched upon in the discussion of mitral valve inflow and diastolic dysfunction, but it bears repeating.

An important nonvalvular flow pattern is *pulmonary venous inflow*. When you have an ambiguous read on the mitral inflow (is that "normal" E-to-A ratio actually *normal*, or is it *pseudonormal*?), then take a look at the pulmonary veins. If they show a blunted S wave, an enlarged D wave, and a large A wave, then that goes along with diastolic dysfunction. The heart is stiff and the atrium is having a hard time pushing blood into the noncompliant ventricle, so the normal inrush during systole is blunted (blunted S wave), more blood rushes forward when the atrium finally does empty (larger D wave), and more blood goes backward into the pulmonary veins during atrial contraction (larger A wave).

Any other nonvalvular profiles that might come in handy?

Yes! Anytime you are wondering about a structure, you can always lay a Doppler across it and see what gives. Especially when you wander up into views of the aorta or other great vessels, you might see a circle or tube and wonder, "Well, what the Sam Hill is that?" If a patient has distorted anatomy (lymphomatous nodes squishing this and that), you can get mixed up with "is that the aorta coming around, or an innominate vein, or what?" Doppler will at least tell you if you have an arterial or a venous wave pattern.

Remember the tricuspid valve? When that has regurgitant flow (as already mentioned above), then you can always interrogate the hepatic vein. Reversal of flow in the hepatic vein is consistent with severe tricuspid regurgitation.

By that same logic, would it make sense to interrogate the pulmonary veins to look for mitral regurgitation? Yes. Systolic flow reversal in the pulmonary veins is diagnostic for 4-plus mitral regurgitation.

Whip that damned Doppler all over the place, it will tell you all kinds of stuff.

IX. Cardiac Anatomy

Imaging Planes

Time to go back to the model and the pie-shaped slice of imaging that comes out of the echo probe.

And time to take another good look at a plastic model of a heart.

These imaging planes tie in with the BIG 20 views of the heart. These are the 20 views detailed in THE ARTICLE on echo (Shanewise et al., *Anesth Analg* 1999;89:870–884). This article and the 20 views detailed therein are the absolute crux of the TEE experience. Photocopy those 20 views and tape them to your TEE machine. Every time you examine a patient, try to get all the 20 views. Get in the habit of "examining everything every time." If not, you'll just look at the "thing of interest" and you'll miss something else.

Also, getting all 20 views will sharpen your TEE probe-wiggling skills. Shanewise gives the lecture on the "standard exam" — meaning the 20 views — and he says he can do it in 7 minutes, before the patient is even draped!

Shanewise has thrown down the gauntlet. Can you do it that fast?

> **TEST NOTE AND REAL LIFE NOTE**   Know these views cold. Know each structure in each view. Imagine you are learning a new language that has a 20-letter alphabet. These 20 views are the letters of that alphabet.

In each view, note the approximate omniplane angle!

The imaging planes for these views are divided into distinct "layers," though, in reality, you slide gradually from one view to another rather than making jerky quantum leaps.

The planes are upper esophageal, midesophageal, transgastric, and deep transgastric. Each plane takes in a few views, except for the pesky deep transgastric, which takes in just one view.

Here's your new alphabet:

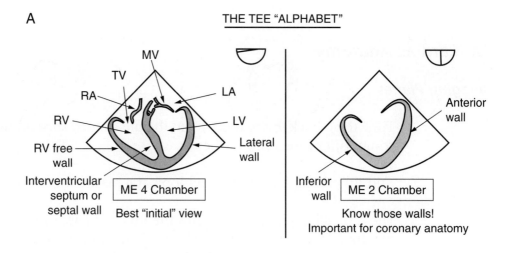

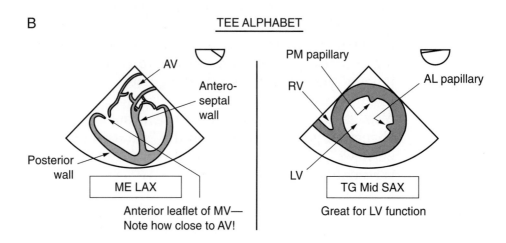

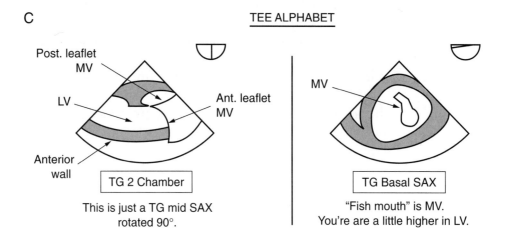

D TEE ALPHABET

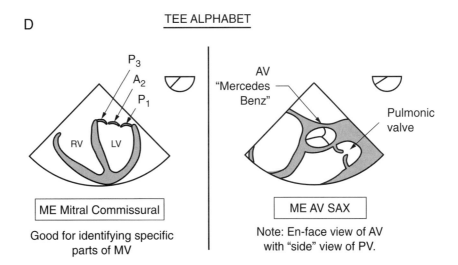

ME Mitral Commissural

Good for identifying specific
parts of MV

ME AV SAX

Note: En-face view of AV
with "side" view of PV.

E TEE ALPHABET

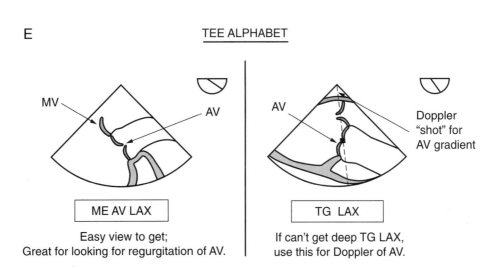

ME AV LAX

Easy view to get;
Great for looking for regurgitation of AV.

TG LAX

If can't get deep TG LAX,
use this for Doppler of AV.

F TEE ALPHABET

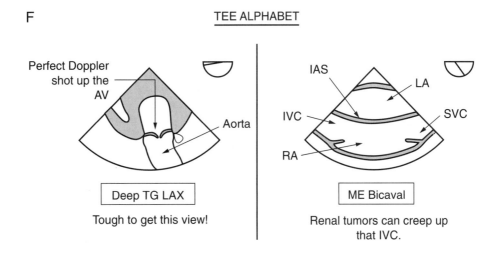

Deep TG LAX

Tough to get this view!

ME Bicaval

Renal tumors can creep up
that IVC.

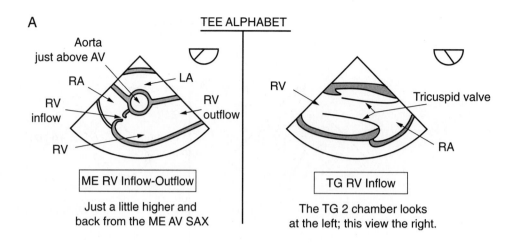

A

TEE ALPHABET

Aorta just above AV
RA
LA
RV inflow
RV outflow
RV

ME RV Inflow-Outflow

Just a little higher and
back from the ME AV SAX

RV
Tricuspid valve
RA

TG RV Inflow

The TG 2 chamber looks
at the left; this view the right.

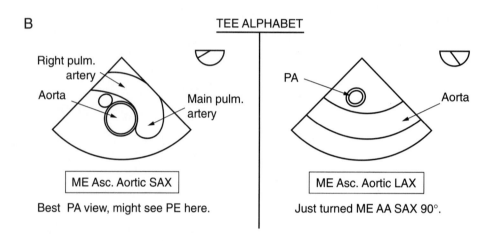

B

TEE ALPHABET

Right pulm. artery
Aorta
Main pulm. artery

ME Asc. Aortic SAX

Best PA view, might see PE here.

PA
Aorta

ME Asc. Aortic LAX

Just turned ME AA SAX 90°.

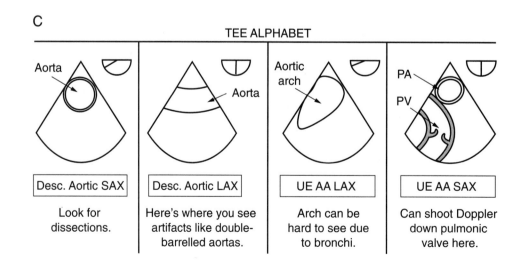

C

TEE ALPHABET

Aorta

Desc. Aortic SAX

Look for
dissections.

Aorta

Desc. Aortic LAX

Here's where you see
artifacts like double-
barrelled aortas.

Aortic arch

UE AA LAX

Arch can be
hard to see due
to bronchi.

PA
PV

UE AA SAX

Can shoot Doppler
down pulmonic
valve here.

DEPOLARIZATION

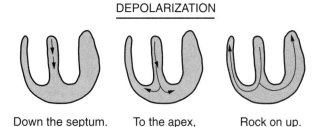

Down the septum.   To the apex,   Rock on up.
                      turn the corner.

Go over these views in detail. Know how to express your findings as related to the views, for example:

"In the bicaval view, I see an ASD."

"In the 4-chamber view, I see a clot in the apex."

"The ME 2-chamber view shows a new regional wall motion abnormality; the inferior wall is not moving."

That's how you want to work with the "TEE Alphabet."

Cardiac Chambers and Walls

The four-chamber view gives you your best "initial impression" and a good look at most of the major stuff in the heart. It's what you first see when you're just starting TEEology.

When you show this view, most medical people can immediately grasp what's going on because it looks like a drawing of the heart. If you have a med student, ICU nurse, surgeon, or someone else looking on, this view shows you all four chambers of the heart (hence the name), the lateral and septal walls, and the mitral and tricuspid valves. What a deal!

And, niftier still, if you just rotate the view 90 degrees, you get the two-chamber view and see the inferior and anterior walls. Rotate 90 more degrees, and you get the long axis view, revealing the anteroseptal and posterior walls. Voila! You've seen all the walls of the heart.

As time passes, you'll get to know what each view can "do" for you.

Now go transgastric, and you see all this stuff in cross section.

This systematic look at the walls of the heart will help us later when we study coronary anatomy. (Preview: By knowing which wall you're looking at and which coronary feeds it, you can tell which coronary vessel is not working. IschemZzzia leads to wall motion abnormalities and bingo! You, Sherlock Holmes, MD, will nail the diagnosis.)

Knowing which wall is which seems a little tough at first, but a little brutal memorization early on will pay off handsomely later.

Need a little crutch? Try this.

Draw a cross section first and get those walls down. Then, draw lines connecting each to its opposite wall. That will get you to link these walls in pairs and keep you from getting mixed up.

"WALL PAIRS" IN CROSS SECTION

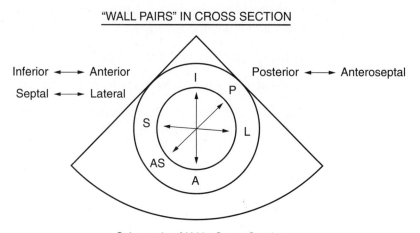

Inferior ←→ Anterior
Septal ←→ Lateral

Posterior ←→ Anteroseptal

Schematic of LV in Cross Section

We will break these walls down further into segments later on, in Section XIV (Segmental Left Ventricular Systolic Function) of this outline. But before you can know the wall *segments*, you need to know the *walls themselves*, so work on just that for now.

Cardiac Valves

Back to Med School for a minute.

> The mitral valve is between the left atrium and the left ventricle.
>
> The aortic valve is between the left ventricle and the aorta.
>
> The tricuspid valve is between the right atrium and the right ventricle.
>
> The pulmonic valve is between the right ventricle and the pulmonary artery.
>
> All valves have three leaflets except the mitral valve, which has two.

Too simple for you? Believe it or not, it's worth reviewing because, in a test or in a hairy case, you *can* and *do* get amped out and go, "Wait, that's the…uh…"

It is comforting to know that there is *nothing* we are incapable of forgetting.

Cardiac Cycle and Relation of Events Relative to ECG

Again, this is Med School redux, but it's worth rehashing to make sure you have it all down ice cold.

Break it down into sections. Since it's a "cycle," you can start wherever you want.

Let's start at the *P wave* of the EKG.

Atrium contracts, blood flows through the mitral valve into the left ventricle. And on the right side? Atrium contracts there, too, and blood flows from the right atrium into the right ventricle. Is more going on? Well, yes. There is some backward flow into the pulmonary veins at the time of atrial contraction, too. And on the right side? Does it make sense there might be a little backward flow there too? (There are, after all, no valves to prevent it.) Yes, by golly, there is a little backward flow there, too, into the two "feeders" of the right atrium, the inferior and superior venae cavae. Should there be a little backward flow down the coronary sinus? That, too, lacks any valves to prevent backward flow. My guess (I never read this or heard it mentioned in any lecture) is yes.

God all fishhooks, Batman, all that going on just with the stupid P wave. I thought this section would be simple!

On to the *QRS complex*.

First, recall how the electricity travels through the ventricle.

As the ventricle depolarizes, the ventricle contracts, slamming the mitral and tricuspid valves shut, and opening the aortic and pulmonic valves.

Oh, that was easy, not nearly so complex as that damned P wave.

Now, the *ST segment*.

After the ventricles are done contracting, the aortic and pulmonic valves close, and the ventricles continue to relax (isovolumic relaxation) until the pressure falls so low that the mitral and pulmonic valves can open and start filling the ventricles.

That's what goes on with the heart itself. It's worth taking a second look at this stuff. This time we'll look at the CVP and the SGC and review what goes on and when.

All those descents and letters and stuff are a pain in the ass, no doubt. (Sort of like the Kreb's cycle; you memorize it a few times in school, then promptly forget it after the test.) But, alas, the docs giving the TEE review course went over these more than once, so it looks like you have to learn it again.

A *wave* — pressure increases from atrial contraction

X *descent* — in systole, as the ventricle contracts, the atrium is sort of "pulled down" and the pressure decreases

V *ascent* — venous blood flows into the atrium, increasing the pressure

Y *descent* — the tricuspid valve opens, pouring blood into the right ventricle and decreasing the pressure in the right atrium

What makes this interesting, of course, is when things go wrong. Regurg, stenosis, congenital malformations, all kinds of things can throw that waveform off. But you have to know the *normal* wave to make sense of the *abnormal*.

X. Pericardium and Extracardiac Structures: Anatomy and Pathology

Pericardium and Pericardial Space

There's a significant "Duh" factor associated with the pericardium. You can be looking so carefully at the *heart itself* that you forget to look *around* it. So you are looking for wall motion abnormalities, valvular function, septal this, pulmonic that, and then someone will ask, "What about that thick ribbon of dark all the way around the heart? What about that 10-gallon pericardial effusion?"

Oops! Damn! You're right.

So if there is one easy take-home, take-to-the-test lesson about the pericardium, just remember to *THINK ABOUT THE DAMN THING*, and you'll probably see what you need to see.

You can see right atrial systolic collapse and right ventricular diastolic collapse with tamponade. Why?

In *systole*, the pressure in the right *atrium* is lowest, so the pericardial effusion can squish the right atrium.

In *diastole*, the pressure in the right *ventricle* is lowest, so the pericardial effusion can squish the right ventricle.

PERICARDIAL EFFUSION

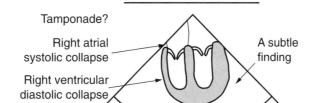

Tamponade?

Right atrial
systolic collapse

A subtle
finding

Right ventricular
diastolic collapse

Pericardium

REAL WORLD NOTE   Back to the stuff you use every day. When someone goes to hell in a handbasket in the OR or the ICU, you place the probe and look for THE things that the echo can tell you. The things that will give you the quickest answers. The things that mean life and death right now:

- Heart empty or full

- Heart beating well or beating badly

- Tamponade

You don't need to be echo certified, echo testamunted, echo expert even. At a glance, most people with minimal echo knowledge should be able to tell these things. Tamponade (of interest in this part of the outline) is, of course, a *clinical diagnosis aided by the finding of a pericardial effusion.* Tamponade is not an "echo diagnosis."

At the TEE meeting they bring up pericardial findings a lot during the discussion of trauma. No surprise, since tamponade occurs so often after car wrecks, stab wounds, gunshots, and other gruesome things.

In the trauma patient, the TEE is especially useful because a transthoracic look at the chest is often impossible. Chest tubes, bandages, sub-q air, and the like make a "frontal attack" on the heart impossible, but a "from the back" look at the heart quite possible. Keep in mind though, in penetrating trauma, the contraindications to TEE, to wit:

Esophageal pathology

Esophageal trauma

Make sure the knife-and-gun club didn't tear the esophagus. You don't want to place your probe and convert a slight rent into a complete disruption of the esophagus.

A zinger in the "normal anatomy that fakes you out" department is the many weird folds and twists of the normal pericardium. The transverse sinus is a great faker-outer.

A pericardial effusion looks like a big black area around the heart. It looks like, well, it looks like a pericardial effusion! Usually even the dimmest medical student in the room can see and identify the fluid-filled sac around the heart. This is no great intellectual leap you need to take here. Just think about it and you'll see it. Things can get a little tricky if the effusion is stringy or gummy (called Wrigley's Double Mint syndrome), but the idea is the same: too much fluid outside the heart.

A little tougher is telling the difference between tamponade and restriction (call restriction a kind of "hardened tamponade") on the mitral inflow patterns.

(Confession time: I've wrestled with this thing and never quite got it. They just seem like the same thing to me. With any luck, you're smarter than I am and really get it.)

Otto (p. 225), has a great table of how to tell pericardial tamponade from pericardial constriction from restrictive cardiomyopathy. Damned picky, testable stuff, and damned hard to get down, too. (You could spend hours on it and still get the test question wrong, so I recommend you just look it over, then either hope they don't ask it or else you guess lucky.)

Pulmonary Arteries

Look at the views that give you your best shot at seeing the pulmonary arteries:

- ME AV SAX — shows the pulmonic valve and the very beginning of the pulmonary artery

- ME RV inflow-outflow — just a tad higher than the earlier view, showing maybe a little more of the PA

- ME asc aortic SAX — best shot of the PA, showing it going up and around the aorta

- ME asc aortic LAX — just a 90-degree turn of the earlier shot, now showing the PA *en face*

- UE aortic arch SAX — a good down-the-pipe shot of the PA, allowing you to do Doppler studies

All these are in the TEE Alphabet. Look at those drawings and cover up the labels. Make sure you can identify the PA in each view. While you're at it, cover up *all* the labels and make sure you can identify everything. Get a sketch pad and draw them yourself. Make sure you can draw a rough picture of what every view looks like.

Your drawings are bound to be better than mine!

> **TEST NOTE** I don't think I'm revealing any state secrets when I say they may show a picture of one of the Big 20, place an *X* on something, and ask, "What is this structure?"

A principle of ultrasound comes into play with the pulmonary arteries. Ultrasound does not work "through" air. The left pulmonary artery ducks behind the left mainstem bronchus, so you only see the left pulmonary artery for a short distance before it disappears. You can follow the right pulmonary artery farther out.

The biggest pathology problem we might see in the pulmonary artery is pulmonary embolus. Of course it is 4+ neato to actually SEE the embolus sitting plunk, right there in the pulmonary artery.

> "Hmm, an *embolus* sitting in the *pulmonary* artery. Could it be, might it be, perhaps, a *pulmonary embolus*?"

There is a kicker here: a pulmonary embolus usually doesn't yield so easily. Most pulmonary emboli are not visible on TEE; you have to see indirect signs of the embolus. (The embolus itself may be so far out that you can't see it, or the *embolus* may be multiple *emboli* "plugging" the pulmonary artery flow by zillions of teeny "pluglets.")

This subject is discussed in a great lecture during the TEE review course entitled "Hypoxemia in the ICU." The notes for that lecture are skimpy, though.

What might you see, then, to show significant obstruction to pulmonary outflow? You might see acute dilatation of the right side in a four-chamber view, with hypovolemia on the left side.

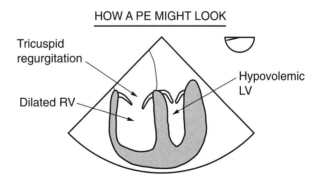

HOW A PE MIGHT LOOK

Tricuspid regurgitation

Hypovolemic LV

Dilated RV

I my very own self saw such a picture in a woman admitted for pulmonary embolectomy. It was quite easy to reason this out.

There is a big plug keeping the right side from emptying, so the right side is "all swoll up," and no volume is able to make it over to the left side, so that side is "all shrunked up."

You might see other signs of "right ventricular struggle":

> If the pressures get high on the right side, you might raise the right atrial pressure enough to pop open a probe-patent foramen ovale.

> High pressures in the right ventricle may cause tricuspid regurg, with backward flow going all the way back to the hepatic veins.

You, the detective, have to put the whole picture together:

- Clinical setup for PE

- Hypoxemia

- Echo findings consistent with a plugged right side

Voila!

You can confirm with a spiral CT scan (of course, don't send the patient off to the dark, spooky, and dangerous confines of Radiologyville if he or she is unstable).

Pulmonary Veins

The Big Kahunas at the meeting say you can see all four of the pulmonary veins. I take my hat off to anyone who can. It's all I can do to see the left upper pulmonary vein. Here's where you see it:

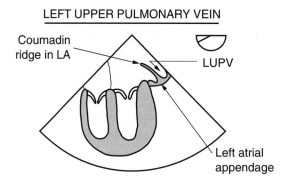

Why bother? With this angle, you can lay a Doppler across it and look for pulmonary vein inflow patterns. Of most practical significance, you can look for systolic reversal of pulmonary vein flow in a patient with mitral regurgitation.

That finding is *diagnostic* for severe, 4+, need to replace or repair the mitral valve, need to do something regurgitation. That makes a real live difference in the real live world.

Do you need to look down the other ones? Not really.

Venae Cavae and Hepatic Veins

Where do you see the venae cavae?

The ME bicaval view is it.

This view can be a little tough to get. It's pretty easy to get a good view of the right atrium, but then you have to "cheat backward" a little to get that view of the inferior and superior venae cavae. A look at the model shows just how "far back" the venae cavae enter the right atrium:

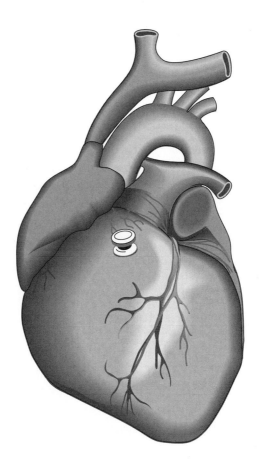

This is jumping the gun, but the venae cavae have a few doodlies to watch out for:

The *inferior vena cava* (on the left side of the screen in the ME bicaval view) can have a confusing piece of anatomy, the eustachian valve. This is seen in 25% of patients, and is located at the junction of the IVC and the right atrium.

The *superior vena cava* has a similar thingie, the crista terminalis.

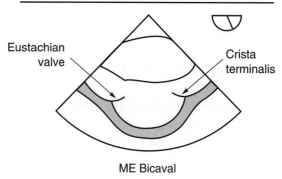

EUSTACHIAN VALVE AND CRISTA TERMINALIS

Eustachian valve

Crista terminalis

ME Bicaval

Both the eustachian valve (IVC) and crista terminalis (SVC) can fake you out and look like a thrombus or tumor.

The hepatic veins you have to hunt for a little. None of the "Big 20" are dedicated to visualizing the hepatic vein, so you have to make your own view. Place the probe deep and turn it away from the heart. You'll see a stippled thing with some big vessels going through it. That's it, you've got it.

The liver looks like…well…the liver. The only thing that could fake you out might be a collapsed clump of lung.

Of hemodynamic significance, you can lay your Doppler in the hepatic vein and look for systolic flow reversal to indicate severe tricuspid regurgitation.

Coronary Arteries

The TEE is not going to let you see much of the coronaries themselves. The TEE is *great* at showing you wall motion abnormalities, which show the *result* of coronary occlusion, spasm, or kinking, but you won't see much of the coronaries themselves.

Here's one view that will at least show you a little — the ME AV SAX:

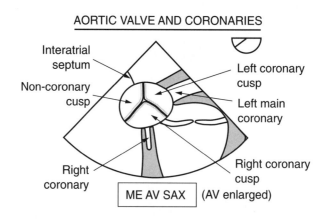

AORTIC VALVE AND CORONARIES

Interatrial septum

Non-coronary cusp

Left coronary cusp

Left main coronary

Right coronary

Right coronary cusp

ME AV SAX (AV enlarged)

Note the three labeled cusps of the aortic valve. The noncoronary cusp is next to the interatrial septum. The left coronary cusp (on the right of the screen — remember, you're looking at a *prone* patient) gives rise to the left main coronary. The right coronary cusp (toward the bottom of the screen) gives rise to the right coronary artery.

In my drawing you see these coronaries, but in real life you may not.

In some circumstances, you can lay a Doppler across the left main. It's damn good to see some flow there!

For thrills and chills, sometimes you can "follow" the left main for a while and see the division into Circ and LAD. This doesn't have that much real significance, but does elicit a few "oohs" and "aahs" in the OR.

In the ME AV LAX and the TG LAX, you might be able to snag a view of the coronaries too, but that doesn't have much real clinical significance. Conceivably, these could be starred on a test with a "what is this?" question tagged on.

Section XIV includes a subsection called Coronary Artery Distribution and Flow. That information is major league important both in real life and in a testing setting. That section is worth knowing ice cold.

Here's a preview of what you should know. (In the TEE review course, they had an entire nighttime review session on this very subject.)

- The posterior wall is not moving; which coronary is involved? (Circ)

- The anterior wall is akinetic; which coronary is involved? (LAD)

- In this cross-sectional view, which wall is not moving and which coronary is involved?

- In this ME two-chamber view, which wall is not moving and which coronary is involved?

That is what you really need to know about the coronaries. Direct visualization is not so important.

Aorta and Great Vessels

> **REAL WORLD NOTE**   This is the scariest aspect of being *"The TEE-Doc"* in the middle of the night. Ascending aortic aneurysms are scary in the best of circumstances, and have a nasty tendency

to occur in the tiny hours of the morning when there may not be "someone else" around to help you read the echo. So you're already spooked at a patient with a BIG PROBLEM. You may be trying to isolate a lung, stabilize a patient, and get some monster lines. And now you're trying to answer the question, "Is there an aneurysm?" and "Where does it start?"

Plus, maybe the patient has lots of other problems (car wreck victim with lots of other trauma; CAD patient whose chest pain *may* be coronary ischemia or may be ischemia *plus* a dissection or may be ischemia *due to* the dissection — ay Chihuahua!).

And the crowning glory? High aortic views are rife with artifacts. And lots of those artifacts *look like* dissections. The very person who is likely to get a dissection is the person who has a lot of calcification, which leads to artifacts up the whazoo.

Woe betide the TEE-Doc facing an ascending aortic dissection.

Anatomy

We have lots of views of the aorta — ME LAX, ME AV LAX, TG LAX, ME asc aortic SAX, ME asc aortic LAX, desc aortic SAX, desc aortic LAX, UE aortic arch LAX, and UE aortic arch SAX.

Go ahead and look at them in the TEE Alphabet. Make sure you can identify the aorta in each view. (Note how often you read, "Make sure you can identify…" The TEE is there for you to IDENTIFY stuff, after all.)

To examine the aorta along its length (which is what you really want to do in that all-important "Is there a dissection?" situation), get the ME AV LAX view and "walk up the aorta," pulling the TEE out a little as you keep the aorta in view.

The aorta has three layers (back to histology land), the tunicae intima, media, and adventitia. The media is the meat of the matter, the tough stuff. Dissection occurs between the intima and the media.

That's the *microscopic* anatomy of the aorta.

The *macroscopic* anatomy of the aorta presents some headaches.

The curvy course of the aorta makes it tough to follow as it winds through the chest. It curves up and over the pulmonary artery, and then follows a somewhat baffling series of twists and turns as it goes through the chest.

Atherosclerosis

Grab a Big Mac, super-size those fries, and wash it all down with a triple-thick shake. Time to lay a little atherosclerosis on that aorta. Back to basics — atherosclerosis lays grunge along the inside of the vessels. TEE is great at picking this up.

This is of big-time significance to aortic cannulation. (For years, surgeons have palpated the aorta to "tell" when there is serious calcification. Their fingers are inaccurate and insensitive. Epiaortic echo, laying an echo right on top of the aorta, is much better at "seeing" atherosclerotic goombas hiding just below the aortic cannulation site.)

AORTIC ATHEROSCLEROSIS

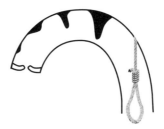

Progressively More Ominous

These monsters get graded. Like always grade 1 is no big deal and grade 5 is a big killer wobbling thing just ready to break loose and wreak havoc.

Aneurysm

Whereas *dissection* is the separation of the intima from the media, an *aneurysm* is an outpouching of the whole Magilla; all three layers balloon out. Marfan syndrome is a classic cause of aortic aneurysm, with a host of other causes (hypertension, cystic medial necrosis, atherosclerosis, trauma, collagen vascular and inflammatory diseases).

Aneurysms can occur in weird places, like the sinus of Valvalva right at the beginning of the aorta. Such an aneurysm looks like a wind sock.

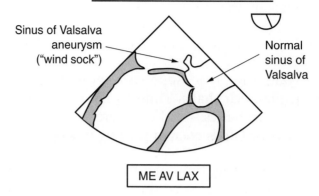

SINUS OF VALSALVA ANEURYSM

Sinus of Valsalva aneurysm ("wind sock")

Normal sinus of Valsalva

ME AV LAX

> **REAL WORLD NOTE**   These things can be monstrous. When the surgeon opens the chest, consider the case the same as a redo. That is, the aneurysm can be so big that the aorta is just under the sternum. Opening the sternum can also open the aorta, so have blood in the room and have that blood checked.

When the surgeon goes on pump and opens the aorta, take a look at the aortic valve. It can stretch out to the size of a saucer. Most impressive!

Surgeons will be interested in the aneurysm's size, so use your calipers and you're in business.

AORTIC ANEURYSM (e.g., MARFAN'S)

Other structures get distorted

Not hard to imagine an aneurysm going on to dissection

ME AV LAX

Dissection and Traumatic Injury to the Aorta

> **NOTE TO READERS**   You can write VOLUMES about dissections. It's worth reminding yourself at this time that you are going through a *checklist* in a *study guide*, not an exhaustive treatment of all things aortically dissectionotic.

This is the big Daddy mentioned at the start of this section. This is the hairiest clinical situation you will find yourself in with the echo. Other stuff is important, yes, no doubt, but the "is it a dissection or not" issue is a killer. Surgeons may operate inappropriately on a nondissection ("Oh well, it's just a median sternotomy.") or delay inappropriately on a real dissection (high mortality and morbidity) based on the echo findings.

From a stress-to-you standpoint, this is the *stat C-section* of the echo world.

According to one of the Emory cardiologists in the TEE meeting, the best initial view to look at the aorta is to see the aortic valve in the Mercedes sign view (ME AV SAX), then come back to about 120 degrees and start "walking up" the aorta. You'll be looking for a flap.

Artifacts can fake you out.

To "de-artifactualize" the view, think for a minute. An artifact is some aberration from a calcified object or an artificial object (a Swan-Ganz catheter can throw a "dissection-like" reflection). So change the view, change the angle, change something. If the object is real, a different view will still reveal the object. If the object is "virtual," a different view should make it disappear.

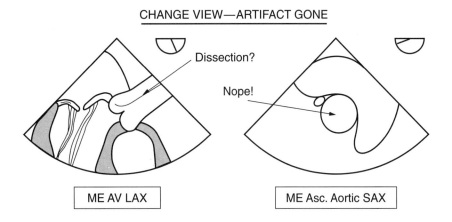

CHANGE VIEW—ARTIFACT GONE

Dissection?

Nope!

ME AV LAX

ME Asc. Aortic SAX

Another good way to tell real from fake is to put the color on. An artifact "ignores" the color flow. A real object will show different flow in the real lumen and the false lumen of a dissection.

A traumatic injury, especially from a deceleration car wreck, tears the aorta where it's "anchored" to the ligamentum arteriosum. So you'll see the dissection when you turn the echo probe around to look backward at the descending aorta. Dissections up in the aortic arch can be a beastie to see on TEE as you are up near the trachea and left main-stem bronchus. You may lose your image to air interference.

When dissection occurs, look for other headaches that can occur with a dissection. The tear can go so proximal that it gums up the works at the aortic valve, causing regurgitation. You can also get bleeding into the pericardium and tamponade.

A dissection starts where it wants and ends where it wants.

The bastard.

Pleural Space

Speaking of bastards, the pleural space is just that. No view in the Big 20 has the pleural space in mind. The pleural space is bound to appear somewhere on the test, as some flagged thing that makes you say, "Hmm, what the hell could that be?"

So how will you know that bunny when you see it?

A pleural effusion on the left side will be seen posterolateral to the descending aorta. That can be a little hard to peg, truth to tell, because the descending aorta follows a kind of curvy path, and you can get faked out as to just where posterolateral is!

An isolated space above the right atrium may also be pleural fluid. But here, again, you may get faked out and think it's pericardial fluid.

Making life even a little more of a headache is this: occasionally, you may get an image of a collapsed lung (looking a lot like the liver) in the pleural space. Oh man!

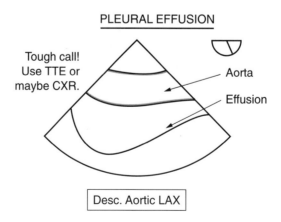

PLEURAL EFFUSION

Tough call!
Use TTE or
maybe CXR.

Aorta

Effusion

Desc. Aortic LAX

My advice? Make sure you know pleural space when you see it. Make sure you can identify the transverse sinus when you see it. If anything else weird shows up, guess pleural effusion and hope to God this one question doesn't determine whether you pass or fail.

XI. Pathology of the Cardiac Valves

Acquired Valve Diseases

Endocarditis

A lot of this stuff lends itself to the second part of the test, the written part. Textbook definitions of things. Pathology discussions. Not really "movie" question stuff. Later (under Tricuspid Valve, Pulmonary Valve, Mitral Valve, and Aortic Valve below) you'll get back into pictures and movies. (Here's where reading Otto's book helps a lot.)

Remember back when we were talking about tamponade and pericardial effusions? Tamponade is a *clinical* diagnosis *supported* by echo findings of a pericardial effusion. But no echo "shows" tamponade.

Same deal with endocarditis. Echo findings of schmutz on a valve *support* a diagnosis of endocarditis, but the diagnosis itself hinges on fever, blood cultures, and a history.

Although they're picky and sort of "Internal Medicine-y," you might want to go over the Duke criteria for endocarditis:

DUKE IN A NUTSHELL

- Pathologic criteria — grow or ID the stuff from the heart lesion itself.
- Clinical criteria — Need 2 major criteria, or else 1 major and 3 minor criteria, or else 5 minor criteria. (Seems like "voting" on a diagnosis but, hey, like I'm going to tell a bunch of ID specialists from Duke how to run the show.)

    Major criteria

        Blood culture of a typical organism

        Evidence of endocardial involvement, such as echo finding or new regurg

    Minor criteria

        Predisposition such as IVDA or predisposing heart condition

        Fever

        Vascular things such as emboli

Immunologic things such as rheumatoid factor or glomeru-lonephritis

Blood culture of a not-exactly-typical bug

Echo finding but not quite as "Aha!-ish" as a major criterion

Whoa, that's enough Internal Medicine Boards for today.

When you look over a patient with real or suspected endocarditis, be sure to look over the *other* valves. It's not a huge stretch to imagine that the same infective process that "soiled" one valve can just as easily soil another one.

> **REAL WORLD NOTE** I had a patient for MVR for endocarditis, and on close inspection of the aortic valve, found a goombah on the aortic valve and we ended up replacing that too.

It would be cool to say that endocarditis looks like *this* and you'd know it's endocarditis. One problem: lots of things can look like lots of things — an echo blob can be a thrombus or infective endocarditis or a noninfective thing (such as Libman-Sacks endocarditis). The view in the echo can't make that diagnosis for you. You have to go with such ancient but reliable technology as a history to help make the call.

A typical lesion, though, is an irregularly shaped mass usually on the upstream side of the valve. Size can vary from teeny tiny to knock your socks off (greater than 3 cm — which spooks hell out of you because you can imaging that monster breaking off and sending an embolus God knows where).

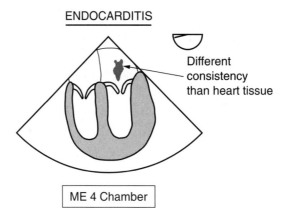

ENDOCARDITIS

Different consistency than heart tissue

ME 4 Chamber

Keep in mind, when looking at any "lump," that you can get fooled. Recall that the echo gives you a 2-D image of a 3-D reality. So, for example, you may think you are seeing a lump on the aortic valve when you look *en face* at the valve. What you are actually seeing is the surface of the regular valve just "coming up" into the picture, then ducking back down out of the plane of the image.

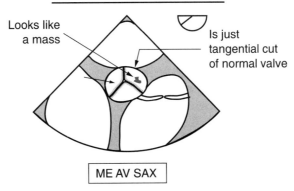

Look at any lump in more than one angle to make sure you're not seeing a figment of your own fertile imagination.

Rheumatic Disease

Why a strep infection should give you this bizarre wipeout of the heart valves is beyond me, but there you have it. Rheumatic disease occurs most often in the mitral valve, but can occur in other valves. Rheumatic disease is the leading cause of mitral stenosis — the leaflets of the valve fusing, thickening, and calcifying:

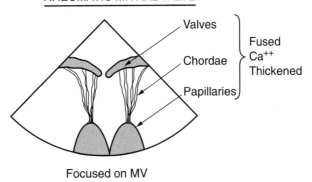

In the aortic valve, too, the valve leaflets fuse, calcify, and thicken:

In Chapter 3, we will look at Doppler signals through stenotic valves.

Do any more valves suffer at the hands of rheumatic disease? Yes. Tricuspid stenosis can occur from rheumatic disease, but in nearly all cases it occurs in conjunction with mitral rheumatic disease. As before, the pathology is the same: the leaflets fuse, calcify, and thicken.

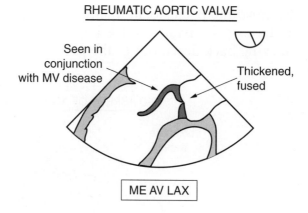

In all these fused, thickened, stenotic valves, the leaflets may bow out (they can't open well, so you can imagine the blood bending the valve as it attempts to open it).

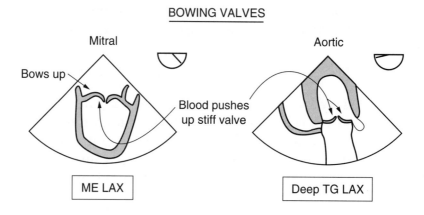

Myxomatous Degeneration

In the mitral position, myxomatous degeneration causes sagging of the leaflets into the left atrium during systole. The leaflets and chordae are thickened and redundant. The disease can be no big deal — mitral valve prolapse but the valve remains competent — or progress all the way to flail leaflet segments with valvular regurgitation.

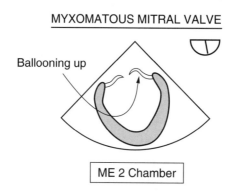

In the aortic position, this same loosey-goosey myxomatous degeneration can occur, causing aortic regurgitation.

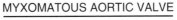
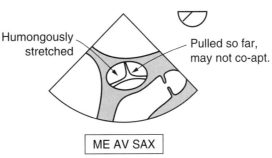

MYXOMATOUS AORTIC VALVE

Humongously stretched

Pulled so far, may not co-apt.

ME AV SAX

Calcific/Degenerative Processes

As we get old and crunchy, our valves do the same. The aortic valve, in particular, takes a hell of a beating throughout its lifetime, so, no surprise, the aortic valve can get calcified and degenerated as we slip into "the golden years." (The calcified years?)

At first the leaflets develop focal thickening, which then becomes generalized. Calcification starts at the perimeter of the valve, then marches inward toward the leaflet's free edges. (Recall that rheumatic disease, in contrast, starts with *commissural fusion*. The degenerative process starts at the *outside* and works inward.)

The right coronary cusp is targeted the worstest, for reasons known but to higher powers. (That's the kind of pimpy thing that might appear on a written test, though, you might want to note.) The leaflets look like they're all encrusted with barnacles of calcium. Depending on just what position they get stuck in, you may get stenosis or a combo pack of stenosis and regurgitation.

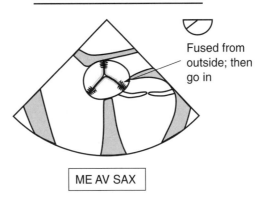

DEGENERATED AORTIC VALVE

Fused from outside; then go in

ME AV SAX

Trauma

(This is kind of freaky if you think about it, but here goes.)

Water is incompressible. If, by some God-awful timing, you get hammered on your chest right at the exact moment all your valves are closed, the shock through the blood (think *depth charge hammering a submarine*) can actually tear a valve leaflet or two. Such a mishap is called the "water hammer" effect. On echo you'd see a perfectly good valve (no calcification, thickening, or other things associated with rheumatic disease, myxomatous degeneration, or calcification) but a leaflet would be torn loose, leading to regurgitation

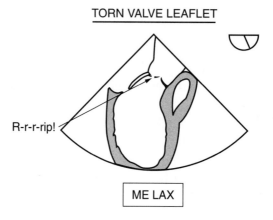

TORN VALVE LEAFLET

R-r-r-rip!

ME LAX

Now, of course, a "water hammer" can also occur to a diseased valve too. What nasty luck that would be.

And if the knife-and-gun club is displaying *fantastic* precision, you could see valvular damage of any shape or stripe, depending on what was used and where it went. There must be some major cool echoes of this kind of stuff. Let's imagine one:

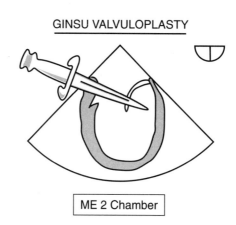

GINSU VALVULOPLASTY

ME 2 Chamber

Tricuspid Valve

What afflicts our friend, the tricuspid valve? Well, lots of things, from endocarditis (the first heart valve that injected bugs "see" is the tricuspid, so, the tricuspid gets gunked up), to carcinoid syndrome (some bizarre chemicals spilling off a GI tumor and "landing" on the tricuspid and pulmonic valves), to fen-phen valvulopathy (no clue how this happens either).

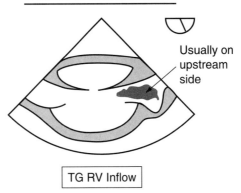

TRICUSPID ENDOCARDITIS

Usually on upstream side

TG RV Inflow

The most common cause of regurgitation is, well, nothing. That is, even a normal tricuspid valve can have some small degree of regurgitation. Lay a Swan or a pacemaker across the valve, and that, too, can cause some regurgitation.

The biggest cause of bad regurgitation (and it's hard to quantify this) is RV dilatation leading to poor tricuspid coaptation. The valve itself is OK, but the RV gets so distended from COPD or pulmonary hypertension that the valve just can't come together well.

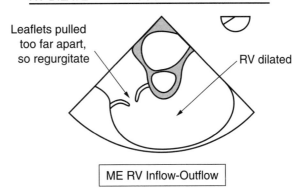

RV DILATE → TRICUSPID REGURGITATES

Leaflets pulled too far apart, so regurgitate

RV dilated

ME RV Inflow-Outflow

There are indicators of TV regurg severity, as listed below (this is from the TEE review course syllabus, first book, page 122):

- Jet area: >10 cm square

- Jet area/right atrial area: >67%

- Vena contracta width: >6.5 cm (The vena contracta is the narrowest portion of the regurgitant jet.)

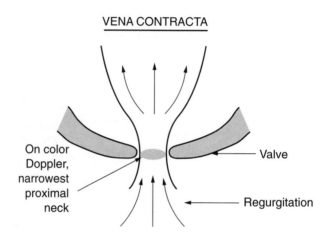

- Hepatic vein flow profile: systolic flow reversal

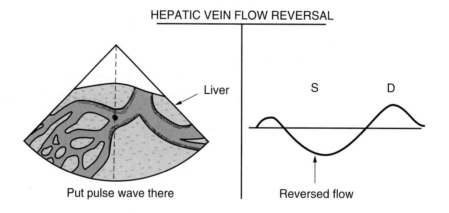

Going on to other indicators of TR severity:

- TR jet intensity: >65% of antegrade flow

- TR jet deceleration: rapid

- TV annular dimension: >34 mm at end systole

But there's a kicker here. You can look at all this stuff, and still be stuck with the question, "So, well, do we replace the valve or not?" Or, "Do we do a valvuloplasty or not?" Also, once a patient's under anesthesia and in a different physiologic state, the regurg may diminish. Oy vay, such headaches!

Having been in the OR when these questions get debated, I can tell you, there is no one answer that will absolutely convince you to go one way or the other. The best you can do is provide the info. Not the world's most satisfying solution, I know.

How about tricuspid stenosis? The most common cause is rheumatic disease.

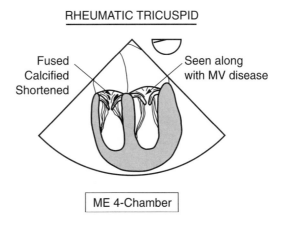

RHEUMATIC TRICUSPID

Fused Calcified Shortened

Seen along with MV disease

ME 4-Chamber

Carcinoid can also cause stenosis, with the valves getting thickened and retracted. Usually severe tricuspid regurg occurs, but stenosis can also be present. The valves get stuck half-open, half-closed, and can't really open or close well.

Rheumatic disease, too, can give you this half-open, half-closed, regurg-stenosis combo pack. The leaflets thicken and retract, the commissures fuse, the chordae fuse and retract too. What a mess.

You can lay a Doppler across the tricuspid and read a gradient.

A mean gradient of 7 mm Hg indicates severe TS, and a gradient of 2 to 6 mm Hg indicates moderate TS, but even this has an "alleged" aspect to it. The gradients are dependent on flow, so if the valve has a lot of regurgitation, then when the blood turns around and goes through the tricuspid valve the right way, you may read a high gradient. But the gradient is just from the high flow, not from any stenosis. So you get faked out! Damnation.

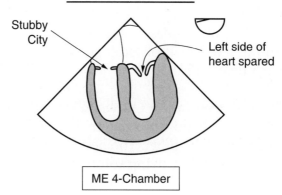

CARCINOID TRICUSPID

Stubby City

Left side of heart spared

ME 4-Chamber

Pulmonary Valve

It's easy to get good views of the mitral, aortic, and tricuspid valves, but the pulmonic can be a bear. Go back to the model to see again how far away the pulmonic valve is from the probe.

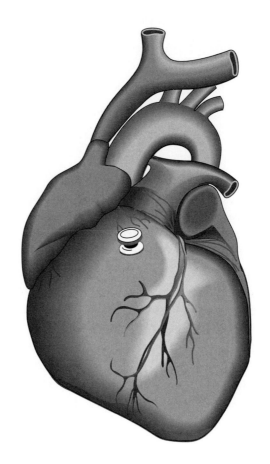

Just as the number one cause of tricuspid valve regurg is "backup" through a dilated RV, so also the number one cause of pulmonic regurg is "backup" from pulmonary hypertension. COPD or heart disease leads to high pressures downstream, and the pulmonic valve (which has a little regurg even when things are *normal*) becomes incompetent.

Remember that list of things that determine *tricuspid* incompetence? Well, no such luck with the pulmonic valve. You can look at the jet height relative to the right ventricular outflow tract (as the author of the lecture at the meeting does), but no one has actually developed a quantitative method of determining pulmonic regurg. You're left with winging it and drawing a kind of qualititative conclusion: "Yeah, it looks bad," or, "Naa, not that bad."

How's that for science?

Rheumatic and carcinoid disease can both cause stenosis (the valves half-open, half-closed again) of the pulmonic valve just as they cause the same problem in the tricuspid valve.

You can get a little quantitative here, using your Doppler to look at gradients. If the peak gradient is

>65 mm Hg, you have severe stenosis

30–64 mm Hg, moderate stenosis

<30 mm Hg, mild stenosis

These valves with their gradients, areas, and such lend themselves in a BIG WAY to test questions. Those kinds of questions appear in Chapter 3.

Mitral Valve

Mitral Regurgitation

> **REAL WORLD NOTE** As surgeons more and more do mitral valve repairs, and get away from replacements, you will get asked a lot to look at the mitral valve for regurgitation. At the meeting, surgeon after surgeon stressed that "physiology is geometry," and a lot of research is going into "remodeling" the heart to make it work more efficiently. There are lots of funky ways surgeons do this, but the bread-and-butter maneuver is repairing the mitral valve by "cinching it up" to prevent regurgitation.

> **TEST TAKING NOTE** The mitral valve, laying closest to the echo probe, lends itself to a lot of test questions. For me (and for others I talked with), one of the hardest things to get down is this: Which section of the anterior leaflet (A1, A2, or A3) or the

> posterior leaflet (P1, P2, or P3) is showing in a given view of the mitral valve? Even scouring the syllabi, you still come up with statements like, "In this view, on the left of the screen you'll see either A1 or A2, depending on the angle." Then on the test, you're stuck, because they give you A1 as a possibility and A2 as a possibility, but not "either A1 or A2, depending on the angle."

Here's what I came up with, but truth to tell, you may want to come up with your own way of tackling this difficult-to-nail-down, sure-to-be-on-the-test question.

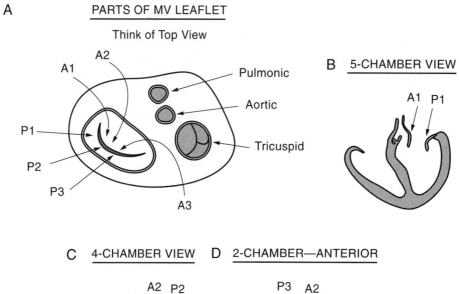

A   PARTS OF MV LEAFLET

Think of Top View

B   5-CHAMBER VIEW

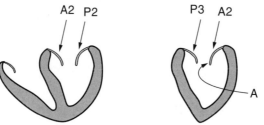

C   4-CHAMBER VIEW   D   2-CHAMBER—ANTERIOR

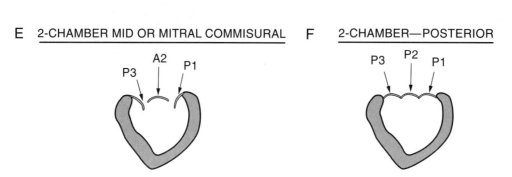

E   2-CHAMBER MID OR MITRAL COMMISURAL   F   2-CHAMBER—POSTERIOR

Easiest view!

Note: In all 2-chamber views, see P3.

Now on to mitral regurgitation.

To get karma-like about the mitral valve for a little bit, let's go back in time. In days of yore, mitral regurgitation meant "that's a bad valve; let's tear out the bad valve, put in a good valve, and bingo, we've fixed the problem." No more complicated than pulling out a bad carburetor and putting in a good carburetor.

Completely interchangeable, no big deal.

Of course, there was the small detail that patients died like flies. Oh well.

Look again at the model of the heart.

The mitral valve isn't just a carburetor that you can yank out. The valve leaflets connect via tough chordae tendineae, which in turn connect with the thick papillary muscles, which then connect to the meat of the ventricle. The mitral valve isn't this *separate*, component part; rather the mitral valve is an *integral* part of the heart. Cutting all those tendineae and wrenching out the mitral apparatus is like cutting all the guy wires that hold up a gigantic radio antenna. Sure, you haven't affected the actual *steel* of the radio tower, but all the supporting parts are gone, and the tower will fall down.

Understanding the *integral, middle-of-everything* nature of the mitral valve will give you a better understanding of all the things that can cause regurgitation.

Anything, anything at all connected with the mitral valve, can make the valve fail, since everything is connected. To see this, start at the left ventricle itself and "work your way up" to the valve leaflets themselves.

- *Left ventricle* — If the ventricle dilates from, say, cardiomyopathy, then the leaflets may get so stretched apart that they can't come together.

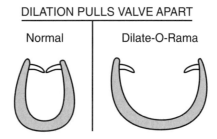

DILATION PULLS VALVE APART

| Normal | Dilate-O-Rama |

- *Papillary muscles* — (Technically, this belongs in the next section, but what the heck.) If these fail, from, say, ischemia, then the connection of the chordae tendineae fails and the mitral valve leaflet may become flail.

ZAP THE PAPS

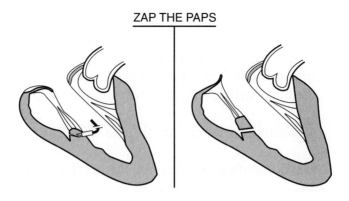

- *Chordae tendineae* — Back to the guy wires analogy and the radio tower. If these connections go, then the leaflet comes loose.

CLIP THE CHORDAE

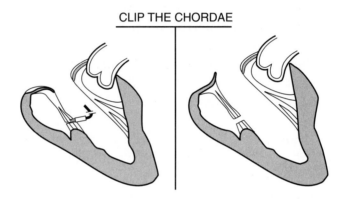

- *Valve leaflets themselves* — Rheumatic heart disease can gum up the valves, as can endocarditis, trauma, you name it. If the valve leaflets themselves fail, then, of course, you can get regurgitation.

LEAFLETS THEMSELVES

Normal

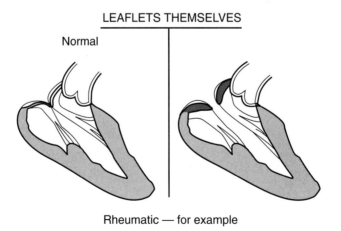

Rheumatic — for example

Picture that mitral valve with all its connections, and you'll be able to peg mitral regurgitation.

Ischemic Mitral Valve Dysfunction

OK, OK, we could dwiggle the semantics here and say, "Ischemia leads to overall ventricular dilatation and that leads to the mitral valve not coapting and you get mitral regurg from that."

What a stretch.

What they're getting at here is, specifically, ischemia leading to papillary muscle dysfunction leading to mitral regurg. In its most extreme form, ischemia can lead to a complete rupture of the papillary muscle.

Which papillary muscle is at most risk for ischemia?

The posteromedial. This papillary muscle usually has a single-vessel blood supply. The anterolateral papillary muscle, in contrast, has a double blood supply, so it is less likely to get ischemic.

Damn, that's a good question type thing and NOT that hard to memorize. I hope they ask you that!

A complete papillary rupture is often fatal, so we tend to see partial ruptures, or a weakening from ischemia, leading to valvular insufficiency.

It's worth reviewing, at this point, that the function of the papillary muscles is NOT to contract and open the valve; rather, the papillary muscles keep the valve leaflets from going backward.

Mitral Stenosis

Thank God for small favors, you don't need to know a million causes of mitral stenosis. Rheumatic heart disease is THE cause of mitral stenosis. Valves thicken, calcify, and fuse, and the chordae tendineae suffer a similar fate.

OK, I lied. I said there was only one cause for mitral stenosis.

But, well, there is another cause.

Mitral annular calcification can also cause mitral stenosis.

Sorry. I wanted to make it simpler for you. It won't happen again.

It's worth knowing the numbers on stenosis, because you can study the holy Bejeebers out of the mitral valve, get all kinds of numbers, and make a reliable call. (Recall the opposite end of the spectrum — the pulmonic valve, too far away to make reliable measurements.)

Normal valve area: 4–6 cm squared

Significant stenosis: 1–1.5 cm squared

Severe stenosis: <1.0 cm squared

Fatal stenosis: 0 cm squared

Chapter 3 will take you through the flaming hoops of quantitative mitral stenosis stuff.

Systolic Anterior Motion of the Mitral Valve

This is cool the first time you see it in real life, no kidding.

Back to the heart model. Look at just how big and long the anterior leaflet of the mitral valve is. It almost hangs down like a curtain.

Think, now, of your shower curtain at home. When you turn on the shower real high, that makes the pressure in front of the curtain low, and the curtain is "sucked" forward.

Same deal happens with the anterior leaflet of the mitral valve. If the anterior leaflet is too big and redundant, or if the septum is too thick, then the distance from the anterior leaflet to the septum is small.

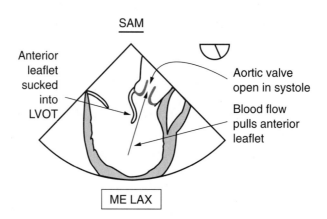

Then, as blood rushes out of the LVOT, the "curtain" of the anterior leaflet is "pulled forward," just like the shower curtain at home. The anterior leaflet of the mitral valve then obstructs outflow.

Treatment?

Get the anterior leaflet (the shower curtain) farther away from the outrushing flow of blood (the stream of the shower). So the simplest treatment is just plain old volume. That will fill and open up the ventricle, separating the leaflet from the LVOT and "breaking the suction."

Of course, surgical repair is another option: either resecting the septum (if the patient had hypertrophic obstructive cardiomyopathy) or cinching up the mitral valve.

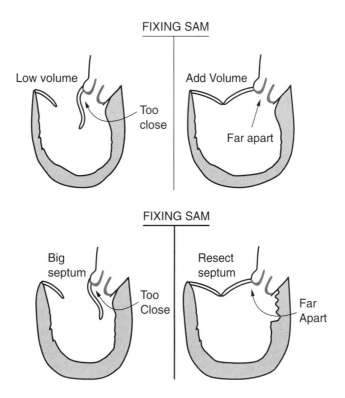

Aortic Valve

Aortic Regurgitation

The aortic valve, cheek and jowl next to the mitral valve, is also easy to see, easy to study, and thus easy to generate lots of questions from.

> **REAL WORLD NOTE** When a surgeon is thinking about doing a *mitral* valve repair, he or she will want a good, good look at the aortic valve, looking for any signs of regurgitation, before and after the operation. The surgeon knows that yanking, suturing, and adjusting the mitral apparatus may alter the aortic valve (they share the same structural ring, after all).

The surgeon has another reason for asking. If the aortic valve is regurgitant, then the antegrade cardioplegia will not work. The cardioplegia solution will all go back through the incompetent aortic valve rather than down the coronaries.

If the aortic valve is regurgitant, then the surgeon will need to place a retrograde cannula to achieve good cardiac quietude.

To understand aortic regurg, take the "holistic approach" we've used with all the other valves. Yes, valve damage itself can lead to valve dysfunction (duh), but other things can gum up the valve apparatus. Most significantly, aortic dissection going down into the valve, or an abscess distorting the leaflets, can prevent coaptation. Also, aortic dilatation can pull the leaflets farther and farther and farther apart, until the leaflets can't come together.

Here are a few pictures to illustrate:

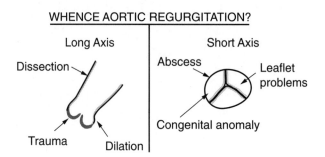

Here are a few more lists (lists are a pain in the ass, no doubt, but they're the kind of things that might appear on the written part of the test).

INTRINSIC VALVE PROBLEMS

- Rheumatic heart disease (in any discussion of the heart, rheumatic heart disease keeps coming back, like an ex-spouse's lawyer)

- Calcified and myxomatous stuff

- Endocarditis

- Congenital defect

- Trauma

ASCENDING AORTA PROBLEMS

- Dissection from trauma or hypertension

- Cystic medial necrosis

- Moldy stuff (sounds more jovial than "mycotic aneurysm")

- Marfan syndrome

Here's a not-too-hard, might-be-on-the-test thing to know. Lay a Doppler in the aorta. If you see holodiastolic retrograde flow in the *proximal* aorta, you have aortic regurgitation, but you have to see holodiastolic flow reversal in the *abdominal* aorta to diagnose *severe* aortic regurgitation.

Repeat:

> Holodiastolic flow reversal in the abdominal aorta is diagnostic of severe aortic regurgitation.

> Holodiastolic flow reversal higher up? Not specific to *severe* aortic regurgitation, it just tells you that there *is* regurgitation.

You can also use continuous-wave Doppler to diagnose the severity of aortic regurgitation. Figure below shows what should be obvious: with severe regurg, the blood flow drops off quickly (the blood rushes back into the heart through the regurgitant valve). With not-so-severe regurg, the blood flow doesn't drop off so quickly.

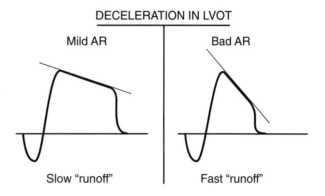

Chapter 3 will tell you the quantitative stuff.

Aortic Stenosis

Sick to death of these valves yet? Fear not. We're on the last valve, last lesion. Plow through this, then pour yourself a cold one.

Bicuspid valves account for most stenosis.

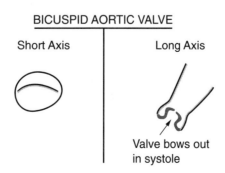

Look for systolic doming. The valve can't open, so it gets pushed out by the force of systole.

Just as other valves can get stuck "half-open, half-closed," so also with the bicuspid aortic valve. Then you get the familiar combo pack of aortic stenosis and regurgitation.

Rheumatic disease causing stenosis at the aortic valve? Sure. It does it everywhere else, why not here?

Calcific degeneration can also lead to stenosis. The aortic cusps start fusing at the outside edges and move progressively inward. This is in contrast to rheumatic disease, which starts at the tips of the cusps.

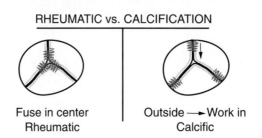

RHEUMATIC vs. CALCIFICATION

Fuse in center
Rheumatic

Outside ——► Work in
Calcific

Once the valve is all calcified and fused, it would be hard to say with great certainty, "Aha, that is typical rheumatic, and this is typical calcific degeneration."

At the meeting, they made a big deal about measuring the aortic valve area. (In the real world, once they've decided to do an aortic valve replacement, they just cut open the aorta, stick in a sizer, and place the appropriate size. No surgeon has modified the size of his or her valve based on my arithmetic.) But from a take-the-test point of view, you need to know this stuff.

Planimetry doesn't work in the calcified, degenerated valve. The three-dimensional outlet can be so tortuous and irregular that picking one 2-D view and measuring with a drawn outline is just no good.

Doppler gradients and the continuity equation are better for getting the aortic valve area. Check out Chapter 3 for all the gruesome detail.

XII. Intracardiac Masses and Devices

Tumors

REAL WORLD NOTE   It's rare that you will be the first one to see a tumor in or around the heart. But you may get called into an OR (particularly during a renal cancer resection) to see if the tumor has crept up the IVC and might be peaking into the right atrium.

Myxomas are the most common primary tumor of the heart. Most often they're attached to the interatrial septum and project into the left atrium. Less commonly, they stick into the right atrium. They're jolly little puppies, bouncing around in the atrium (sometimes occluding the mitral or tricuspid valve, which can take some of the jollity out of the room in a hurry). As they bounce around, everyone in the room is sure to "ooh" and "aah."

TEE can be such a blast sometimes!

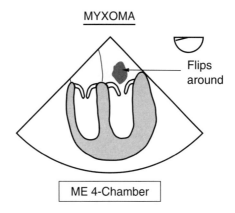

What's cool about myxomas, too, is their curability. Zing! Out they go, everyone goes home happy.

Less groovy are rhabdos, which tend to invade the wall of the ventricle. A rhabdo is, after all, a muscle cell gone haywire.

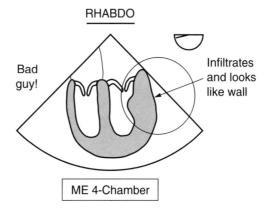

When it comes to secondary tumor masses and where they can go, the sky's the limit. Any cancer can take up residence in the pericardium, the transverse sinus, the lung with extension wherever, the pleural space (remember, the pleural space can be hard to identify; now put a distorting tumor in it and you're lost), or mediastinal nodes.

(On the test, you've just got to hope they'll have an easy-to-identify myxoma.)

This gets into the material in Section XVII (Artifacts and Pitfalls), but it's worth looking at now.

Pectinate muscles, the Coumadin ridge, and developmental leftovers can mimic masses. Thrombi (see the next part of this section in the outline) can also mimic tumors.

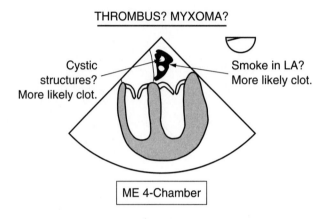

The interatrial septum can develop something that looks, to all the world, like some God-awful infiltrative process. Lipomatous hypertrophy of the interatrial septum makes the septum look like a barbell, with the narrow part being the fossa ovalis.

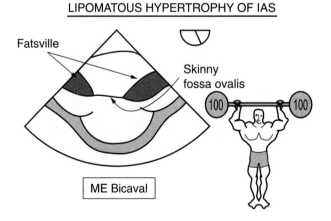

That won't get you the "oohs" and "aahs" of a good myxoma, but people will think you're cool because you know it, so practice pronouncing it a few times so you come off slick.

Lipomatous hypertrophy of the interatrial septum.

Yeah.

Thrombi

Left atrial enlargement and/or atrial fibrillation can lay the low-flow groundwork for a left atrial thrombus. The low flow shows up as "smoke" in the TEE.

Once the clot has formed, it can attach to the atrium or even bounce around free, like a big beach ball floating above a marijuana-impregnated Grateful Dead concert.

Attached, a thrombus can look a lot like a myxoma.

At the meeting, this "which is which" came up a few times, and there's no foolproof way to know for absolute sure. Here again, history would help.

Cystic stuff clues you in to thrombus formation, but, then again, could a myxoma not break down in the middle, leaving a little cyst in it? Sure.

As in the previous discussion of tumors, certain developmental things and regular anatomic things can throw a "spanner in the works":

- Coumadin ridge

- Eustachian valve

- Chiari network (a lacelike network floating around in the right atrium, attached to the eustachian or thebesian valve at one end and the crista terminalis or atrial wall at the other)

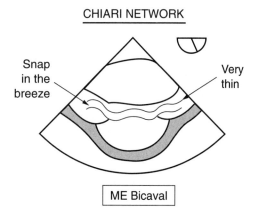

CHIARI NETWORK

Snap in the breeze

Very thin

ME Bicaval

- Crista terminalis

While we're on the topics of thrombi, don't forget that all thrombi do not occur in the atrium. The ventricle can get a big old thrombus at the site of an MI.

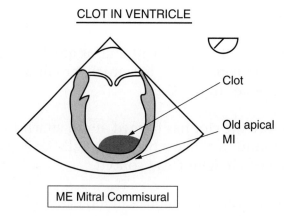

CLOT IN VENTRICLE

Clot

Old apical MI

ME Mitral Commisural

Could a thrombus be *outside* the heart? Sure. In a creepy scenario, the heart itself could bleed into the pericardium, the patient could somehow survive, and a clot could form there. In the trauma arena, a mediastinal bleed could also lay a clot around the heart.

Here's a little spooky tidbit from our criminal justice history. Some group did MRIs on people who had been legally hanged. They didn't see broken necks. Instead, they saw big mediastinal bleeds, so it looked like the convicted criminals died of tamponade rather than from a snapped cervical vertebra. I got this from my old roommate, a radiologist privy to such eerie information, so I guess it's true.

I didn't ask whether they did TEEs on the guys.

Devices and Foreign Bodies

The headache of "this is a 2-D image of a 3-D reality" becomes a reality with all the catheters, wires, and junk we stick in patients. Swans dip in and out of view. Groshongs, dialysis catheters, even monster catheters like left-ventricular assist device drainage catheters are forever diving into view and dipping out of view. The plastic coating can throw shadows, too, creating artifacts.

> **REAL WORLD NOTE**   Mentioned before but worth mentioning again: If you are worried about aortic dissection, have a Swan-Ganz catheter in, and are concerned about whether an imaged line is an artifact or a dissection, pull the Swan out and take another look.

A catheter usually has a "dual-line" appearance.

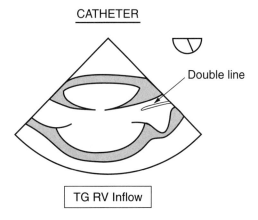

Any catheter can have a thrombus or infected vegetation.

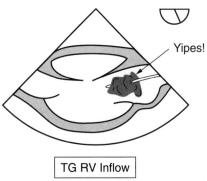

Foreign bodies can be whatever cruel, cruel mankind decides to place into his fellow man. Myself, I like how we refer medically to "missiles" when we're talking about bullets.

I mean, missile, you picture a Titan V rocket sticking out of the poor guy in the ER.

XIII. Global Ventricular Systolic Function

Normal Left Ventricular Systolic Function

> **REAL WORLD NOTE**   If you're just getting going on echos, try to see as many echos as possible. Just poke your head in the cardiac room and sneak a peak at every echo done in your ORs. Noting normal function is a lot easier after you've seen a lot of normal echos. (This comes from the DUH Institute of Common Sense.) More than any quantitative measure, normal ventricular function is a Gestalt call.

A surgeon at the meeting pointed out some interesting stuff about the ventricles. When we imitate the heart with our fist, we squish our fist shut. But the ventricle doesn't work like that. The left ventricle moves more like a piston, with the apex holding still (look at a beating heart in the cardiac OR if you don't believe me) and the mitral ring area moving down.

The shape of the heart is important, too. A normal left ventricle is shaped like a football. That allows an efficient ejection — a spiral pass — to go far downfield. (Versus a dilated heart, which looks like a basketball. You can't throw a basketball as far as you can throw a football.)

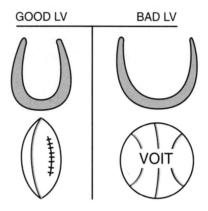

If you want to get more systematic about this, you can measure the fractional area of the left ventricle using a true long- or short-axis cross section:

$$\frac{\text{End-diastolic area} - \text{end-systolic area}}{\text{End-diastolic area}}$$

You outline all these areas, you try to align just right so you get a "true" long- or short-axis view, and you let the computer spit out the data.

Or — what really happens — you just look and go, "looks like crap, that's a 20% EF."

On the test, you might not be able to "eyeball" the difference between 25% and 32%, but you should be able to tell 30% from 50%. The practice tests on the CDs will help you tell this.

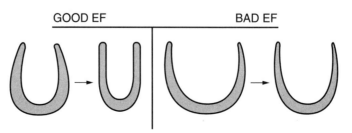

Abnormal Left Ventricular Systolic Function

Etiologies, Including Ischemia

OK, um. One etiology is ischemia.

Wow, wasn't that easy?

Going through the causes of global left ventricular dysfunction is kind of an "oral boards in anesthesia" exercise. One method is to start at the outside and work your way in:

- *Pleural space* — Tension pneumothorax squishes off the blood vessels, no venous return, no perfusion, no ventricular function. I sure as hell hope you don't need a TEE to diagnose a pneumothorax.

- *Pericardial space* — Tamponade can result from pericardial effusion or pericardial blood. TEE is major groovy for helping make that diagnosis.

- *Ventricle itself* — Infiltrative disease such as amyloidosis can cause global impairment.

- *Empty ventricle* — This is a bit of a stretch as a cause of global hypokinesis, but what the heck, we're trying to list all the causes of left ventricular dysfunction.

- *Ischemia* — We already said that.

- What's *in* the blood — Global ventricular dysfunction can certainly occur due to "bad blood": hypoxemia, hyperkalemia, hypoglycemia, anemia — pick your metabolic poison.

Assessment of Ejection Fraction

This hearkens back to the previous discussion of Normal Left Ventricular Systolic Function in this section. Most TEE folk eyeball the EF.

Confounding Factors

Positioning is everything, as they say to all newlyweds, and so it goes with reading an accurate EF. If your attempt at getting a "true" long- or short-axis section of the left ventricle is off-true, then you won't get an accurate read.

Another kicker is the problem of regional wall motion abnormalies. If you look in one "slice" and the ventricle looks spiffy, you may assume the whole ventricle is spiffy.

TANGENTIAL SLICE OF LV

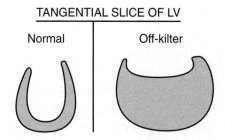

Normal   Off-kilter

But noooooooooooooooooooooooooooooooooooooooooooooo!

Another slice may be awful. So be sure to take a few different views.

Right Ventricular Systolic Function

Back to the model of the heart.

The *left* ventricle is pretty compact, regular shaped, and easy to quantify, even with your eyeball. Not so the right ventricle, a "C"-shaped thing that kind of wraps around the left ventricle. No one panoramic view allows you to take it all in, so you have to settle for a qualitative, rather than a rigorously quantitative assessment.

One thing that helps is (believe it or not) something mentioned by a surgeon at the meeting. Whereas the left ventricle is a piston, with the whole mitral structure moving down as one, the right ventricle has a kind of "hinge" motion.

RV AS HINGE

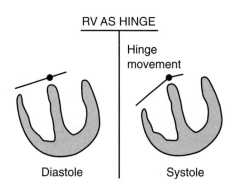

Hinge movement

Diastole   Systole

Looking at the corner of the tricuspid valve move gives you a good idea of how the right ventricle is working.

In the four-chamber view:

- The RV should be triangular and should only extend about two thirds of the length of the LV. If the RV goes farther, you have RV hypertrophy.

- The end-diastolic area of the RV should be no more than 60% of the LV.

- The apex should be made by the LV. If the RV makes the apex, bad news.

- The overall shape of the RV should stay triangular. If globuloid, you got trouble, right here in River City.

Another view that is useful for looking at the RV is the RV inflow-outflow view, which goes by the snappy moniker "wraparound view," since the RV wraps around the aortic valve.

Keeping that aortic valve in view helps keep you looking at the right ventricle. (You can get goofed up looking for this view and end up seeing the "RA inflow-outflow view" — that is, the bicaval view — by mistake.)

Another thing to look at is the septum. RV hypertrophy can lead to paradoxical septal movement — the interventricular septum pushing over to the left.

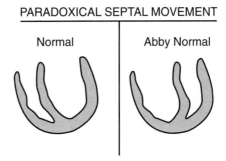

PARADOXICAL SEPTAL MOVEMENT

Normal   Abby Normal

Now here comes a pimpy, detailed-enough-to-be-on-a-test factoid:

Volume overload (ASD, tricuspid regurg, pulmonic regurg) leads to septal distortion maximum at end *diastole* — the maximal *volume*.

Pressure overload (pulmonic stenosis, pulmonary hypertension) leads to septal distortion maximum at end *systole* — the maximal *pressure*.

That's not too hard to remember; just think about what's happening and it makes sense.

Cardiomyopathies

Hypertrophic

Four different hypertrophic cardiomyopathies exist, not just the most "famous" one: septal hypertrophy leading to idiopathic hypertrophic subaortic stenosis — itself an antiquated term since everyone says "hypertrophic obstructive cardiomyopathy" now. At the meeting, speakers toss out the acronym for hypertrophic obstructive cardiomyopathy — HOCM — all the time. Pronounced aloud, it comes out "Hokum," like some relative of Li'l Abner and Daisy Mae down in Dogpatch.

For the written part of the test, you have to put on your Internal Medicine/Cardiology hat and pound down some hypertrophic cardiomyopathy trivia:

- HOCM is inherited as an autosomal dominant trait with limited penetrance. (Which, if you think about it, is the ultimate genetic cop-out explanation, since anything at all, any pattern of inheritance you could ever imagine, could ultimately be explained as autosomal dominant with limited penetrance.)

- Four different patterns are seen:

  Type I: anterior septal hypertrophy

  Type II: anterior and posterior septal hypertrophy

  Type III: hypertrophy everywhere but the basal posterior wall

  Type IV: apical hypertrophy only

- That bit about sparing the basal posterior wall is important, because hypertrophic cardiomyopathy can look a lot like the next item on the list — restrictive cardiomyopathy — with one exception. Restrictive cardiomyopathy does *not* spare the basal posterior wall.

- The systolic function is usually normal, but the diastolic function is abnormal. Recall the discussion on diastolic dysfunction — the heart can't relax enough to allow good filling during diastole.

- If you lay a continuous-wave Doppler across someone with the classic outflow obstruction, you will see a dagger-shaped outflow pattern, versus the normal rounded shape. This occurs because, during late systole, the ventricle gets so empty that obstruction to flow occurs.

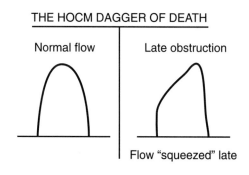

THE HOCM DAGGER OF DEATH

Normal flow | Late obstruction

Flow "squeezed" late

- SAM is a distinct possibility in the setting of septal hypertrophy. The outflow tract is already narrow as narrow can be, so that anterior leaflet of the mitral valve can suck right in there and impede flow.

To relieve this obstruction, decrease contractility (that's why Halothane is the classic anesthetic for this kind of case) or keep the volume up. If, in blazing contrast, you increase contractility or drop the afterload and empty the heart, you'll worsen the obstruction.

Sometimes we jump into the fray here and participate in septal resections. We do an echo before the resection to confirm that the lesion actually exists. (That comes from the DUH School of Medicine — make sure the patient *has* the disease before you perform an open-chest operation to cure that disease.)

After the resection, you repeat the echo to make sure that you resected *enough* septum to relieve the obstruction, but not so much that you created a ventricular septal defect.

To recap:

Take out too little: persistent obstruction

Take out too much: VSD

The conduction system of the heart runs right through this area, so watch that ECG. Persistent heart block can and does occur, so make sure your pacer box has a fresh battery in it when you do one of these septal resections.

We keep an eye out, during this surgery, for complications such as rhythm disturbances (the conduction system is so, so close to where the surgeons are resecting), ventricular septal defects (Oops! Went too far), or persistent obstruction (Oops! Didn't go far enough).

SEPTAL RESECTION

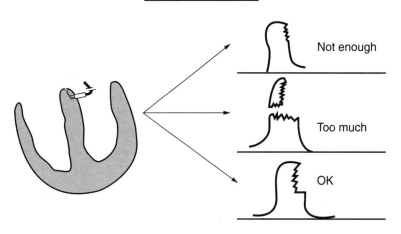

Restrictive

Creepy, rotten things sneaking into the myocardium cause restrictive cardiomyopathy. Amyloid, iron from hemochromatosis, sarcoid, glycogen stuff from those bizarre glycogen storage diseases, and eosinophils from a rare disease called Loffler's endocarditis round out the baddies that cause restrictive heart disease.

As noted above, a hypertrophied, thickened heart from a restrictive process can look a lot like a hypertrophic cardiomyopathy. The only distinguishing feature will be that *spared posterior basal segment*. And, no surprise, our old friend the history and physical may arrive on a white charger and save the day for us.

Here's how they might look side by side:

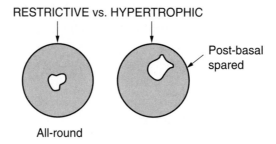

Left ventricular function may hang tough for a while, but diastolic dysfunction (that inability of the ventricle to relax and "accept" good filling) occurs.

Another aspect of this worth remembering is that, with restrictive heart disease, a left ventricular thrombus may occur *without* an underlying wall motion abnormality. This can occur in the apex or under the posterior leaflet of the mitral valve, leading to mitral regurgitation.

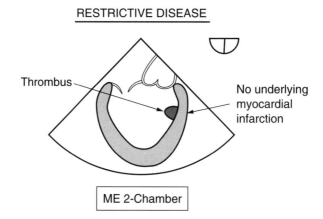

This is a good time to go back and review diastolic dysfunction.

Remember how different maneuvers and how pulmonary vein flow patterns will help you tell the difference between normal and pseudo-normal patterns of LV inflow.

Dilated

This is the diagnosis you peg in an instant when you see the whole heart is all flabby and it looks like all four chambers just gave up.

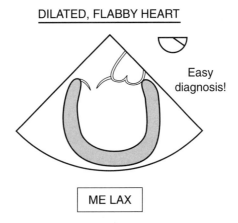

DILATED, FLABBY HEART

Easy diagnosis!

ME LAX

Since nothing much is moving in this heart, clots can form.

Causes of dilated cardiomyopathy? The list is as long as your arm:

- Idiopathic (a perennial favorite when we don't know Jack)
- Postviral (another great yawning abyss of ignorance; how come one cold gives you the sniffles and the next one gets you a heart transplant?)
- Peripartum (ditto)
- Alcohol
- A zillion others

XIV. Segmental Left Ventricular Systolic Function

Myocardial Segment Identification

Hear ye, hear ye. The Office of Homeland Security is not going to shoot me for revealing any state secrets here. You will need to know these segments and you will need to know which coronaries feed which walls and which segments.

I kid thee not.

I speak not with forked tongue.

At the meeting, they lay broad hints on you that this is a *for sure* on the test.

The first time you see it you'll quasi freak, because it looks so complex, but when you think of all the other stuff you memorized to get this far, it's not so bad. Plus there's a logic to it, so don't go off the deep end.

First, the whole thing, then we'll back up and break it down.

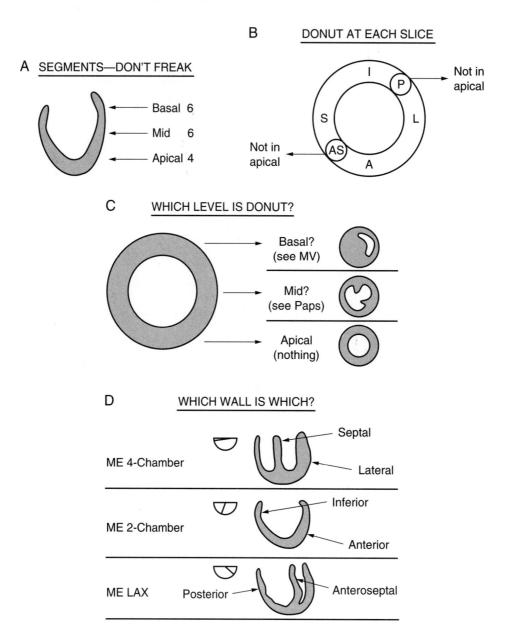

I found it easiest to start with the cross sections. That way you can at least always know what's "directly across" from you. Then you can take the long views and start to put it together.

So, think of three of these laying on top of each other, starting at the top of the ventricle, right next to the mitral valve. Three layers of six:

>The basal 6 segments are next to the mitral valve.

>The middle 6 segments are next down, at the level of the papillary muscles.

>The lower, or apical, 6 segments come next.

BUT WAIT!

Though it would make sense to do 6/6/6, the SCA (perhaps fretting about the demonic number 666 from *The Omen*), only recognizes four segments in the ever-narrowing apex.

Lose the posterior and the anteroseptal segments there. In the apical, you just have inferior, anterior (across from each other, remember), and septal and lateral (across from each other too).

Now, put it back together, piece by piece, until it makes sense.

Coronary Artery Distribution and Flow

REAL WORLD NOTE Major, major importance that you know this. This ties in with the extremely practical dilemma that you face on a daily basis: "Is the new graft working?" If a wall fed by, say, the right coronary graft *was* working, and now *is not* working, hey, look at the graft for kinks, disconnects, clots, dissections. It's a hell of a lot easier to recognize the problem and fix it *now* than to find out later and lose a chunk of myocardium.

TEST NOTE Vintage testable material here, folks. A little brutal memorization (come on, there are only three vessels, it's not that bad) and you should nail these questions. How important is this at the TEE meeting? One of the nighttime sessions is dedicated to this very issue. Everyone but everyone attended.

Pictures tell it all:

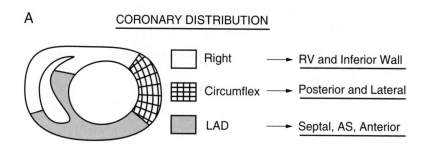

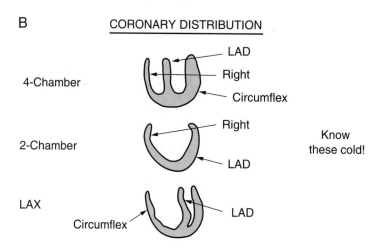

Let's put it into words, just in case you're less of a visual learner.

The *right* coronary feeds the *inferior* wall and *right ventricle*.

The *left anterior descending* feeds the *anterior* and *septal* walls. (No wonder an LAD infarct is so problematic.)

The *circumflex* feeds the *posterior* and *lateral* wall.

Everyone at the meeting studied the hell out of this issue, drawing the pictures over and over again, flashcards, you name it. Get this stuff down but down.

Normal and Abnormal Segmental Dysfunction

Assessment and Methods

Keep your eyes open, that's the method. The wall motion abnormalities you see will *not* be subtle. Every test taker since the dawn of time emphasized that to me.

"You'll see it moving, then BOOM, it ain't moving."

And in real life, that's what you see too. As soon as a wall gets ischemic, the motion disappears. Keep in mind, the normal movement of a wall is thickening and an inward movement.

At the meeting, they get a little more scientific than this, saying "Normal contractility results in 30% thickening of the wall, hypokinetic is 15%, akinetic is, well, 0%, and dyskinetic means it bulges outward."

Others gets a little more Gestalty:

- Normal is normal looking.

- Hypokinetic is hypokinetic looking.

- Akinetic is akinetic.

- Dyskinetic is dyskinetic looking.

Golly.

All of this high-tech ranking is groovy, but you just have to look at a bunch of echos and try to peg, "Which wall is not happening?" This can be harder than it seems, so be systematic about it. Look at one section and (this according to the great Cahalan himself) say, "Systole, systole, systole" and see if *that particular section* moves.

In the OR, I'll put my finger in the center of the ventricle on the monitor and see if different wall segments move in toward my finger.

One trick I stumbled upon is the value of fast forward. Tape a bit, then rewind and look at the walls in fast motion. Believe it or not, when the ventricle's going super fast, the dyskinetic or akinetic wall stands out better than at regular speed.

In your studying, look at either the tapes or the CDs. This is a total "moving picture experience," for there is no other way than to drill these. On the tapes from the 2002 meeting, they recorded the "Regional Wall Motion Unknown" session. That is the best way I found to practice picking out the "mystery wall motion abnormality."

Differential Diagnosis

Well, gee whiz, what else could it be?

Wise counsel says, "Believe bad news and act accordingly." Other than a graft not working or a native vessel being occluded, there aren't too many other things it could be. The main aspect of the differential should center on *which* catastrophe afflicted your graft:

- Air embolus (particularly after an open procedure)

- Spasm of the internal mammary (A surgeon at the meeting and in the tapes points out that spasm of the internal mammary graft is an oft-cited excuse. In reality, the graft was poorly placed, kinked, or clotted off, and the all-encompassing excuse of "Oh, it must have been spasm" is pulled out for public consumption.)

- Too long of a graft, leading to a kink

- Too short of a graft, leading to a squinking shut of the graft as it's stretched flat as a pancake

- Clot from, perhaps, hypotension and stasis (Eeek! That can be a result of "Anesthetica Imperfecta"!)

- Dissection

Whatever it may have been, when you *see* a new wall motion abnormality that you *thought* you should have fixed, take a look-see.

Confounding Factors

Tethering can throw you off the hunt when examining regional wall motion abnormalities.

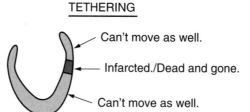

TETHERING

Can't move as well.

Infarcted./Dead and gone.

Can't move as well.

A hypo-, dys-, or akinetic area can "hold back" a normal area. (*You* may be able to run around pretty energetically, but if I jump on your shoulders and say, "Yeehaa! Giddyap!", your motion may slow down considerably. You have been *tethered* by my bulk.)

The angle of your examination may throw you off too. If you get a really foreshortened view of the ventricle, for example, you may not get a clean look at one segment; rather, you'll see a lot of segments at once and won't be able to make a clean diagnosis.

Left Ventricular Aneurysm

An aneurysm is a thinning of the entire wall of a structure. So, on echo, a ventricular aneurysm is seen as a dyskinetic region (bulges outward in systole) that has a diastolic contour abnormality (keeps bulging outward even after systole is over). In other words, the damned thing is always bulging out. Kind of the "love handles" of the heart.

Of specific diagnostic interest, an aneurysm has a *smooth transition* from normal myocardium to thinned aneurysm. There is no sharp angle or neck (as we'll see with pseudoaneurysms or ventricular ruptures in just a minute).

The love handle analogy helps again. Love handles (however much they may plague us, uh, more *mature* gentlemen) at least have an aesthetically pleasing smoothness as they transition from the torso to the love handle proper.

Aneurysms are most often found in the apex, though they can occur elsewhere. And aneurysms, with their underlying stasis, can give rise to thrombi.

Left Ventricular Rupture

For a big-time ventricular rupture, skip the TEE. Grab a pathology text and head for the refrigerated surgical suite in your hospital's basement.

A *survivable* rupture through the myocardium but contained within a "skin" of pericardium is called a "pseudoaneurysm." On echo, you don't see the smooth transition of the true aneurysm; rather, you see a narrowed neck at the site of the breakthrough.

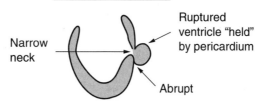

PSEUDOANEURYSM

Narrow neck

Ruptured ventricle "held" by pericardium

Abrupt

If you want to get all quantitative and anal about it, the ratio of the neck to the maximum diameter of the pseudoaneurysm should be less than 0.5. But give me a break; if you know what happened, the difference between an aneurysm and a pseudoaneurysm should jump out at you.

XV. Assessment of Perioperative Events and Problems

Hypotension and Causes of Cardiovascular Instability

> **REAL WORLD NOTE**   Let's face it, cowboys and cowgirls, this is the real crux of the whole deal with echo. All the cool physics and gradients and Doppler stuff are necessary for the test. And if you're going to do cardiac echo, you need to know all the neato-frito valve details. But as TEE gets more and more common, the day will come when every single anesthesiologist or ICUologist will need to know at least the basics of TEE to *figure out what's going on when a patient gets unstable.*

The TEE is the anticrash weapon of choice.

When badness happens, (and we've all seen it happen), you might not have a Swan or CVP. And even if you do, you're still wrestling with numbers that tell you *something*, but not the *whole picture*. You are left with a set of numbers from which you *infer*, or *hope*, you have the picture.

The TEE *gives* you the real picture, right now, no need for a leap of faith.

Cahalan points out in the tapes and at the meetings that, even with only a little TEE experience, most people can diagnose the most common problems in mere minutes. After all, when most patients go to caca, you want to know

- Heart full or empty?

- Ventricle good or bad?

- Tamponade, yes or no?

For most problems, then, Cahalan gives us a nice, neat, easy-to-understand and inherently obvious breakdown of the main causes of hypotension:

1. End-diastolic area decreased, ventricle contracting OK — You're low on volume. The heart is empty, so fill it.

2. End-diastolic area increased, ventricle contracting poorly — You have a bad and already overfilled ventricle. Fix whatever's

causing the global hypokinesis (Get a blood gas! Don't forget the basic stuff!), and once you've fixed what you can fix, it's time for inotropes or ventricular support of some kind.

3. End-diastolic volume normal, ventricle contracting OK — You have a problem with the volume not "going where it's supposed to go." Either the volume is all going out into a vastly dilated circulatory tree (anaphylaxis with low systemic vascular resistance), or else some other channel is misrouting your good cardiac output (severe mitral regurg or aortic regurg, or a ventricular septal defect).

The first two are easy to see with a glance at the TEE. The third is a little trickier, but you can augment your TEE findings with other stuff. (Flushed appearance and wheezing going along with anaphylaxis; murmurs or further TEE views to find mitral regurg, aortic regurg, or a VSD.)

Then the final thing you want to know, "Tamponade, yes or no?", is figure-outable with your basic search for a pericardial effusion plus the hemodynamics of tamponade.

If you take nothing else away from TEE (say you don't want to bother taking the TEE exam), if you at least know this, the differential for hypotension, you will save somebody some day.

Cardiac Surgery: Techniques and Problems

Assessment of Bypass and Cardioplegia

How the hell do you use TEE to assess bypass and cardioplegia? Got me. I have no clue what the Society of Cardiovascular Anesthesia folk were thinking when they put this on their magical list.

Let's stretch a little and try to figure this one out.

Use your TEE to show that the heart is not beating at all – that would mean the cardioplegia is working.

Use your TEE to see that the heart is not blowing up like a basketball — that would tell you that the cannulae are flowing in the right direction and there is not some catastrophic flow reversal.

One thing is worth mentioning at this time. Disconnect your echo probe while on bypass. That will allow the probe to cool down and prevent esophageal burns. And remember that you do need to *disconnect* the probe, not just put the image on FREEZE. Although the word FREEZE implies a cool state of affairs, you have just frozen the *image*. You haven't actually frozen the probe and turned it into a big Fudgecicle.

Cannulas and Devices Commonly Used during Cardiac Surgery

The main cannula you'll be asked to visualize is the retrograde cannula for cardioplegia. First, you need to know where the coronary sinus is (the site of the retrograde cannula).

To see the coronary sinus on TEE, you need to find the interatrial septum, then navigate the probe in a retroflex direction until you can get the entry to the coronary sinus in view. You can do this from the four-chamber view, but you have to cheat over a little bit until you see the right side more.

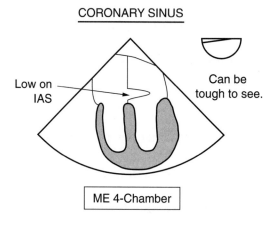

Once you have that dog in view, watch for the cannula to cross the threshold. Like all cannulas, the retrograde cannula has a "double line" that tells you it's a man-made thingamajig. And like all cannulas, its 3-D reality will dive in and out of your 2-D picture, making it sometimes a little tough to keep it entirely in view.

What else might show up during cardiac surgery?

A metallic aortic cannula can throw shadows all over the place. Sometimes I've been asked to look at an aortic valve before decannulation. If the aortic cannula is metal (some are plastic, of course, and don't present such problems), that can make for a tough investigation. The aortic valve is "lost in the noise."

Anytime an aortic cannula is in, a dissection (heaven forbid) *could* occur, so you go ahead and examine the aorta and look for this dreaded complication.

Look at the atrial cannula? Sure, why not? I never do in a routine case and this was never discussed in tapes or at the meeting. I suppose you could imagine looking at the venae cavae if the surgeons were having trouble cannulating, to see if there is a web or some bizarre thing holding them up, but that's a stretch.

Circulatory Assist Devices

It's not a stretch to look for correct placement of an intra-aortic balloon pump. You want to see the tip of the IABP at the takeoff to the left subclavian artery. No higher (occlusion to the left arm) and no lower (inadequate function of the balloon pump).

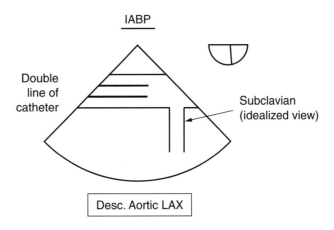

Things can get more exotic, of course.

Left and right ventricular assist devices, and ECMO when things are going really swell, all enter the cardiac realm in this Brave New World we inhabit.

With an LVAD, you want to make sure the person doesn't have a patent foramen ovale or interatrial septal defect. You could, as the blood rushes out of the left side into the assist device, "suck" blood from the right side over to the left.

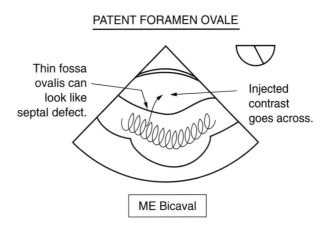

If this happens, then no blood goes out the right side, so no blood goes to the lungs, so no oxygen enters the body. Unless your patient is a cyanobacterium, he or she will need oxygen.

So check for these PFO you start an LVAD.

Once the LVAD is going, you can also use the TEE to confirm that the aortic valve isn't opening.

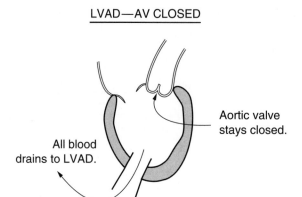

LVAD—AV CLOSED

Aortic valve
stays closed.

All blood
drains to LVAD.

At first that concept seems a little jarring.

"What, the aortic valve isn't opening? But, golly Mr. Wizard, how can the person live?"

Yes, usually that is the case, but remember, you're not in Kansas anymore, Dorothy. The LVAD is doing all the work now. You *want* the blood to all leave the heart and go into the machine.

In testville, remember that the cannula that is draining blood *out* of the body into the machine is the *inflow* cannula. (That is, *inflow* as far as the *machine* is concerned. You could get faked out and think, well, relative to the body, that is technically outflow, so… Don't think that!)

ECMO and RVADs? You can use TEE to check those cannulas too and just make sure they seem to be in the right place.

Intracavitary Air

No biggie here. Air bubbles look like snowflakes swirling around in the heart. You will want to look for these (the TEE is the most sensitive at detecting air bubbles) after an open-chamber procedure to make sure you de-aired the heart properly.

Air can hide out in the tangle of papillary muscles and chordae tendineae. (When you think of a cardiac "chamber," you think of this big, open space, but it's damned crowded in there.) Check along the septum and down in the apex for "lurking air."

Minimally Invasive Cardiopulmonary Bypass

(Perhaps more accurately called "Minimally *done anymore* cardiopulmonary bypass.")

As regular old off-pump CABGs work so well now, the days of MIDCABs (such a puckish name) seem to be numbered. TEE was used to make sure the fantastically complicated tangle of cannulas was all in place.

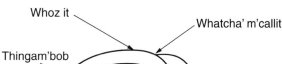

MID CAB CANNULAS

Whoz it

Whatcha' m'callit

Thingam'bob

Reverse transcriptase doodah

Interquark monitor

Thank God this ischemia-producing (in the anesthesiologist) procedure is going the way of the 8-track cassette and the slide rule.

Off-Pump Cardiac Surgery

Now this is more like it.

As a sign of the times, I looked back at the tapes for the 1999 TEE course. People then were talking about doing off-pump cardiac surgery in "select cases" and doing relatively small percentages of people off pump. Well, of course, by now, everybody and their second cousin is doing off-pump CABGs. McDonald's will have a drive-thru window soon where you can get off-pump CABG done.

One pain in the ass, actually THE pain in the ass, with off pumps is "the hike" — when the surgeons lift the heart to get at those dim and distant distals. Hemodynamically the patient's blood pressure often takes a hit with the hike, though the newer "holder thingies" and more surgeon experience have made the whole process less devastating than in days of yore. The hike also goofs up the echo, because now you may have air between the heart and the probe.

No can do the transgastric view, no way.

Hike the heart, the view goes away.

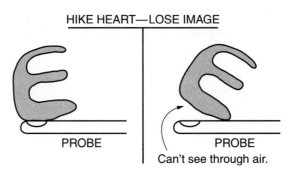

The whole deal during off-pump surgery is, "Can we do this off pump?" or "Are things getting SO BAD that we have to stop this charade, put in cannulas, and do this *on* pump?" Pertinent to us is the question, "Can the TEE help me make that decision?"

What tells you things are going to the dogs?

- Low blood pressure unresponsive to your usual blandishments.

- Ectopy so bad that *you* get ectopy.

- Ditto asystole.

- Rising CVP or PA pressures.

- Increasing mitral or tricuspid regurgitation.

- Regional wall motion abnormalities that persist and persist and (when the hell are they going to finish the graft!?) finally make you and everybody panic and say, "BASTA! The patient's dying! Stop!"

But during off-pump cases, you are actually looking at the wall right there, with your own *eyeballs*. Even "hard to see" walls are hiked up for you and the surgeon and everyone to see. You can, of course, confirm it with the TEE, but your eyeballs do just as well in the OR.

TEE helps you to see the mitral and tricuspid regurg, of course. (Unless you're Superman, most of us can't see inside the heart.)

So how much and how long of a wall motion abnormality is enough to push you "onto the pump"?

Uh…

Jack Shanewise gives this talk at the TEE conference. (He's a great speaker, so don't miss him. Remember, he spearheaded the big paper that gave us the "big 20" views, so he knows from TEE.) He tells us (p. 142 of the second TEE review course syllabus) that at his home base of Emory, they usually see signs of ischemia or wall motion abnormalities during these off-pump cases, but that as long as things improve after the anastamosis is complete, you're usually (not always) OK.

Having heard the talk and done a bunch of off-pump cases, you're still left with a bit of a "by guess and by God" feeling about these off-pump cases:

1. They hike the heart.

2. They clamp the vessels to sew in the graft.

3. Things get bad, you limp along with volume, a little Neo maybe, you hope things don't get *too* bad.

4. TEE confirms that you are limping along, but you hope things get better.

5. Things either get better or they don't.

6. If they don't, if the wall motion abnormality does NOT go away, then you have to reexamine that graft and make sure it's working OK. (If you had an *on*-pump case and had a new regional wall motion abnormality, you would reinvestigate your graft, wouldn't you?)

How's that for the state of the art?

I tell residents an off-pump case is like a labor epidural that's just kind of, sort of working. You pray and pray for the lady to deliver so that you'll just be done with it! Same with these cases: you pray and pray that they get the grafts done so you'll just be done with it!

Coronary Surgery: Techniques and Assessment

How will TEE help you in an *on*-pump CABG? (Since we talked about off-pump just a second ago.)

Pretty much, the TEE will replace the Swan. (This debate will swirl around for a long time, particularly the "What happens when the patient goes to the ICU; do we put a probe in *again* each time we get in trouble? You guys have it in the *whole* time in the OR, but *we in the ICU* don't!")

With the TEE going in nearly all our patients (people at the meeting confirmed that, in a lot of places, heart surgery means a TEE, period), you get most of your "Swan-like" information right there from the TEE. (We *do* put introducers in everybody, so we can always put a Swan in later.)

- Heart empty or full? TEE tells us.

- Ventricle crummy, ventricle snappy? TEE tells us.

- Tamponade? TEE tells us.

In effect, this discussion is the exact same discussion as in Hypotension and Causes of Cardiovascular Instability above. What, after all, are you concerned about during a CABG? Hypotension and cardiovascular instability. So, boom, same exact analysis.

This helps you out at all points of the case. Hypotension and cardiovascular instability can and do happen whenever they want to — at induction, during the IMA dissection, coming off pump, whenever.

TEE also helps in regional wall motion abnormality analysis. This goes right back to another previous discussion in Section XIV (see Coronary Artery Distribution and Flow).

Examine the patient ahead of time, look for wall motion abnormalities. See which grafts go in which distribution. If you see a *new* wall motion abnormality, that is evidence a graft is not working.

This comes in especially handy once the chest is closed. The skin and sternum are "in the way" and the TEE helps you see what your eyes no longer can.

Valve Surgery: Techniques and Assessment

Valve Replacement: Mechanical,
Bioprosthetic, and Other

Not to sound like a broken record here, but TEE helps you during valve surgery the same way it helps you during CABGs, that is, in the evaluation of cardiac function and volumes. The management of hypotension and cardiovascular instability.

TEE helps you keep the blood going round in circles in your patient, and Oh be Joyful to that. How?

- Heart empty, heart full?

- Ventricle good, ventricle bad?

- Tamponade, yes or no?

Do we see a pattern here?

But in valve surgery, we go a little further than management of hypotension and cardiovascular instability. We look at the valve itself, before surgery, to confirm the diagnosis and assess severity, and after surgery, to confirm good function of the valve and make sure there aren't any problems. And yes, once all is done, we go back like dutiful soldiers to evaluating for hypotension and cardiovascular instability.

> **TEST NOTE** You've got a little memorizing to do. You will need to know what different valves look like on echo. Not the end of the world, but the hyphenated double names of the artificial valves drove me cuckoo. Doesn't any *one* person ever design a valve?

Let's plow through the various kinds of valves and how they look. Different ones have different jets of regurg (you'll need to know that too), but one thing holds true for all valve replacements. You should not see a PERI-valvular leak. You shouldn't see leaking OUTSIDE the sewing ring. That means bad news. All valves have some leaking INSIDE the sewing ring, but not, repeat *not*, outside.

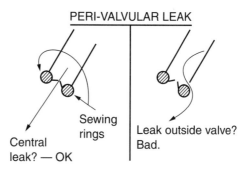

PERI-VALVULAR LEAK

Sewing rings

Central leak? — OK

Leak outside valve? Bad.

Another goody to know: prosthetic valves all need anticoagulation, tissue valves don't. Now, on to the specific valves.

STARR-EDWARDS

Ball-in-cage.

Oldest kind, can last a long time.

Kind of big and clunky, causes a lot of hemolysis.

Since flow goes around the sides, that's where you'll see a couple jets of regurg before the valve closes. (All valves have a little bit of regurg before they close.)

STARR–EDWARDS

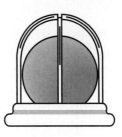

Ball in cage

MEDTRONIC-HALL AND BJÖRK-SHILEY

Tilting disc.

Complex flow pattern.

TILTING DISC

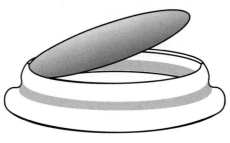

Single Disc

ST. JUDE AND CARBOMEDICS

(Always these double names! At least they settled on just one saint for the St. Jude.)

Bi-leaflet.

Wide open flow helps forward flow, but can lead to a lot of regurgitation.

HANCOCK AND CARPENTIER-EDWARDS

(This really ticks me off, we already have a Starr-Edwards!)

Porcine bioprosthesis.

Has three metallic stents holding it in place, so you still see shadows.

BILEAFLET

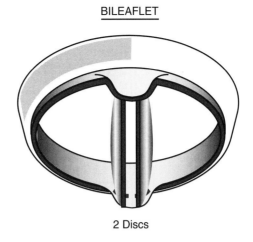

2 Discs

STENTED BIOPROSTHESIS

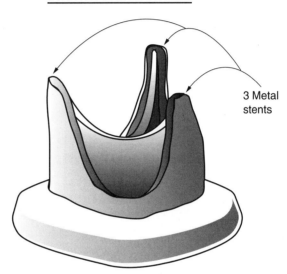

3 Metal
stents

Valve leaflets on stents

ROSS PROCEDURE

Take out the diseased aortic valve, take out the native pulmonic valve, put the pulmonic valve in the aortic place, put a tissue graft in place of the pulmonic valve.

> **TEST NOTE**   For me, the shadows from the tissue valve stents and the shadows from the prosthetic valves can look pretty similar. Watch the video of this or study the CD movies of these a lot because, on the test, you only have a minute or so to look at these, and it can be pretty confusing. If there is one area where you can get fooled, this is it.

There are stentless prosthetic valves. You won't see the metal and their reflections, but you may see a sewing ring. That is an *extremely* subtle finding and easy to miss.

An issue with tissue valves is longevity. They tend to wear out faster.

You can measure gradients across these valves, but it can be challenging. You have to know where the tight spots are and you have to navigate a straight shot through that spot. For example, for a Starr-Edwards, you'll have to slip your Doppler right through one of those regurgitant jets around the sides of the ball.

A useful "Internal Medicine-y" thing to know about gradients: when you are evaluating a valve and see a gradient you think is a little high, remember, *all* valves have *some* gradient. Try to find an *old* reading of the gradient before you ring the alarm bells. The thinking is the same as getting an old ECG or CXR for comparison.

All valves are subject to embolism and endocarditis. So you'll be looking through some confusing reflections (try different angles to avoid the metallic shadow) as you hunt for fistulas, abscesses, and clots.

Valve Repair

Aortic repair?

Doesn't happen too often. A truly isolated injury to one cusp, maybe, but surgeon enthusiasm for aortic valve repairs has faded a bit of late. More often they replace the aortic valve.

Mitral repair?

Now you're talking. This is becoming to cardiac surgeons what appendectomy is to the general surgeon.

First, you evaluate the mitral valve, looking to grade the severity. Four-plus regurg pretty much mandates that "something be done," often a repair rather than a replacement. How do you know it's 4+? Look for systolic flow reversal in the pulmonic vein; that is diagnostic/pathognomonic/for sure for sure, good buddy, that the regurg is severe.

After the repair is done, you will look at the mitral valve again, making sure, well, that the repair worked! Regurg gone (good), but not *so* gone that you have moved all the way to mitral stenosis (not good).

Tricuspid repair?

If the tricuspid valve has severe regurg, you will see reversal of flow in the hepatic veins. (Similar to seeing systolic flow reversal in the pulmonic vein with mitral regurg.) The surgeon may choose to repair it, though they do this a lot less than mitral repairs.

After the repair is done, look for enough repair to stop the regurg (good), but not so much that you have stenosis (not good). Sound familiar?

Pulmonic repair?

Don't see that much, though I suppose you could if you wanted to be really cool.

With all these valves, what might you see that would make you NOT want to do a repair?

Rheumatic, shortened, fused valves do not handle repairs well. Such a valve needs replacement. You want to see a redundant valve, something that gives you something to work with.

Transplantation Surgery

Heart

As far as TEE is concerned, there are only a few special things you'll see with a heart transplant. You'll see extra-atrial tissue and see suture lines that demarcate "the new from the old."

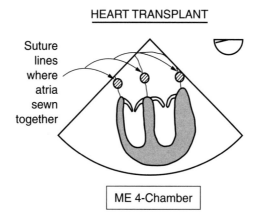

HEART TRANSPLANT

Suture lines where atria sewn together

ME 4-Chamber

From an anesthesia standpoint, one thing you will really be watching for is signs of right heart failure — the big bugaboo of heart transplants. What will you see, by way of review?

- RV enlargement
- Tricuspid regurg

Of course you look for all the usual suspects — hypovolemia, global dysfunction, tamponade — as in every patient. Air, too, can bite you in the butt, but it's the right heart battling against "previously unseen" pulmonary hypertension that will cause the most headaches.

Watch that RV!

Lung

Most lungs are, you sincerely hope, full of air, so it's a toughie to examine them with TEE. So in those rare cases of lung transplants (not done too often or in too many places), you're left with doing the usual stuff — monitoring the heart for signs of failure.

You will yawn when I say this, but you'll be looking to monitor for hypotension and cardiovascular instability; that is, you'll watch for

- Ventricle full or empty?
- Ventricle good or bad?
- Tamponade?
- Valves OK?

What more can I say — by now we keep coming back to the main things a TEE does!

The TEE, your friend indeed in time of need.

Liver

If you put the TEE deep and turn it around, you can look at the liver, though I don't know of many observations you can make. (None were mentioned at the meeting, or in the tapes or any books I read.)

I've been called into liver transplantation surgeries to put the TEE in and look around. Of note, the varices that most of these patients have are NOT a contraindication to placement of the probe.

Truth to tell, there are no special observations to make here either. You use the TEE to monitor hemodynamics (which can be pretty damned exciting in those blood bath/volume-o-ramas). Almost always, trouble comes when you get *behind on volume*, and the TEE reminds us that this is indeed the case.

XVI. Congenital Heart Disease

Take one lesson to *your own* heart in this section on congenital heart disease. Where *one* congenital malformation can occur, *others* can occur. So **do a complete exam on everyone**.

One abnormality doesn't *preclude* another abnormality, and it may very well *presage* another abnormality.

Identification and Sites of Morphologically Left and Right Structures

Those whiffle-ball hearts can send the blood on triple back flips in the pike position, with anomalous return to one side compensated by septal defects shunting stuff to the other side. Then everything gets reversed when the patient gets cold, so who know what goes where.

There is one "trick" that might help you identify what is what: inject fluid in a central line and look for the turbulence on TEE. Wherever the cloud shows up, that is the "right-sided" or "venous" side.

This is a good time to lose your shyness and ask a pediatric cardiologist for help.

Atrial Septal Defects

> **TEST NOTE**   At the meeting they emphasized that you have to know not just that there is an atrial septal defect, but *which kind* of defect it is. Very testable, that.

To get this down cold, take a second to review the normal sequence of events in the development of the atrial septum; then the nomenclature of the defects makes more sense.

First, the septum primum comes down.

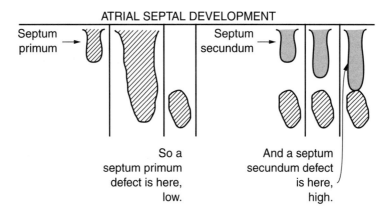

ATRIAL SEPTAL DEVELOPMENT

Septum primum →

Septum secundum →

So a septum primum defect is here, low.

And a septum secundum defect is here, high.

Then the top of the septum primum breaks down.

Then the septum secundum comes down and "flaps over" the septum primum.

Then it follows that a *primum* ASD occurs low down, where the septum primum is.

And a *secundum* ASD occurs a little higher, where the septum secundum *should have* come down. Here is where the fossa ovalis should be, but instead a defect is. (This is also where your probe-patent foramen ovale might be if there weren't a defect already.) This is the most common ASD.

A less common kind of ASD is the sinus venosus ASD, which occurs higher still in the atrial septum.

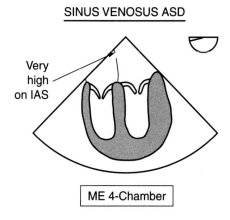

SINUS VENOSUS ASD

Very high on IAS

ME 4-Chamber

Remember at the start of this section how we talked about "one defect indicates another"? Here's a few gems for the ASD department:

- Primum ASD is associated with cleft anterior mitral valve leaflet abnormality.
- Sinus venosus ASD is associated with anomalous pulmonary venous return.

Ventricular Septal Defects

You need to know different kinds of ventricular septal defects too.

Four different kinds here:

- Membranous VSD

    Most common.

    Occurs up high, in the membranous portion of the interventricular septum.

- Muscular VSD

  Can happen anywhere along the muscular interventricular septum.

  Can be multiple.

- Inlet VSD

  The central fibrous body (the "middle of the heart"; the "skeleton" between the atria and the ventricles where the valves are located) fails to fuse. The defect is seen inferior to the aortic valve plane, next to the mitral and tricuspid valve annuli.

  A little tougher to visualize.

  As you can imagine, if the "center" of the heart fails to fuse, other "center of the heart" things can go wrong — primum atrial septal defect (remember, that is real low down), and AV valve abnormalities (they rely on that "skeleton" too).

- Supracristal VSD

  Found in the right ventricular outflow portion of the septum above the crista ventricularis and inferior to the aortic valve.

  Rare.

VSDs and ASDs lend themselves to a lot of gradient-type problems that you'll see in Chapter 3.

Pulmonary Valve and Infundibular Stenosis

TEST NOTE People say the weirder congenital lesions don't appear on tests too much; more often it's the bread-and-butter things such as ASD, VSD, Ebstein's anomaly, persistent left superior vena cava, coarctation of the aorta, and bicuspid aortic valve. Of course, each year they make the test anew, so who knows what will tickle their fancy. From here on there'll be less yackity-yack (as in Section XV above) and more picture recognition.

REAL WORLD NOTE Especially in kiddies, the bizarre flip-flops and rearrangements are, unless you're the most whiz-bang pediatric cardiac anesthesiologist/intensivist, just beyond our ken. Pediatric cardiac surgeons or cardiologists are needed to unravel these mysteries, and a lot of work is done epicardially right in the OR.

Pulmonary Valve Stenosis

Not much to comment on here; the lesion says it all. The pulmonic valve, the exit from the right ventricle, is stenosed. No surprise, then, that you might see signs of right ventricular overload as the "weaker" right ventricle tries to overcome the impedance to outflow.

Here's a diagram of it:

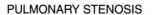

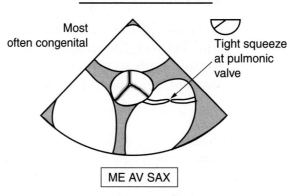

The next lesion just "pushes" the impedance down a little further, right into the right ventricle itself.

Infundibular Stenosis

Sorry, couldn't find any picture of this. But in your mind's eye, you can draw the lesion yourself. The outflow tract of the right ventricle (also called the "infundibulum") is narrowed below the pulmonic valve. (Think of a kind of hypertrophic subaortic stenosis, only now the lesion is sub*pulmonic* instead.)

This lesion is most often due to a long, narrow fibromuscular channel, but can also be from a localized fibrous diaphragm.

If you are torqued up on memorizing, this is also called Dittrich's stenosis. (Named after the famous Belgian cardiologist, Dr. Dittrich Stenosis.)

(Cybernote for all you Internauts — a Google search on any of these lesions yields a plethora of information. My printer just spat out 24 pages on Dittrich's famous stenosis.)

Left Atrial and Mitral Valve Conditions

When they say "left atrial conditions," I think they're driving at cor triatriatum, since that's the only odd "left atrial condition" I've read or heard about.

Mitral valve conditions? Must be cleft anterior leaflet. (Recall that this is seen in conjunction with primum atrial septal defect.)

CLEFT ANTERIOR MV LEAFLET

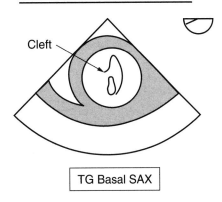

Cleft

TG Basal SAX

Aortic Valve and Left Ventricular Outflow Tract Abnormalities

Aortic Valve Abnormalities

The biggie, biggie, biggie for aortic valves is bicuspid valve. There are unicuspid valves and even quadricuspid valves, but they're damned rare. Knowing of the presence of unicuspid and quadricuspid valves may win you points at some cardiology cocktail party sometime, but knowledge of bicuspid valve will more likely net you some points at a TEE test.

Left Ventricular Outflow Tract Abnormalities

We already looked at HOCM. (As long as you're at that cocktail party, remember to pronounce it "Hokum" and say it a lot. The cardiologists will all think you're hip.) But for congenital stuff, the condition I think they're driving at here is subaortic membrane. A membrane runs from the anterior leaflet of the mitral valve to the interventricular septum, causing obstruction and, counterintuitively, aortic regurgitation!

How does a membrane *before* the aortic valve cause regurgitation? First, the aortic annulus is poorly supported (one defect screwing up the nearby structures). The other reason for regurg takes a little thinking and visualization — there is a high-velocity jet going through the tight orifice of this membrane. The jet is still going, the blood is still "squeezing through," when the aortic valve is trying to close. That "forward jet" keeps the aortic valve from shutting completely.

Sit back for a minute and just digest that, because it takes a little before that settles in your brain.

SUBAORTIC MEMBRANE

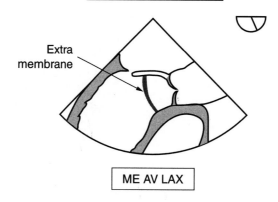

Extra membrane

ME AV LAX

Coronary Artery Anomalies

TEE is not the greatest at visualizing the coronary arteries themselves. Regional wall motion abnormalities? Amen and hallelujah, yes, great great great. But the coronaries *themselves*? More of a curiosity when you do see the takeoff of a coronary. So don't expect any great shakes on TEE detection of coronary artery anomalies.

So what might you see?

Coronary AV fistula. Then, the normally smallish coronary sinus (remember, the collection point for the coronary *veins*) would be dilated because now coronary *arterial* flow would be running into it.

You might also see a larger coronary artery than usual.

I suppose (I'm reaching here) you could see a coronary insert at an abnormal place, say, at the noncoronary cusp of the aortic valve. Some coronaries, after all, don't read the book and do what they are supposed to.

Patent Ductus Arteriosus

Back to embryology. The fetus has to navigate without lungs. One of many features allowing this sleight of respiratory hand is the ductus arteriosus, funneling blood from the pulmonary artery into the aorta, thus bypassing the lungs.

Normally, at birth, the resistance in the pulmonary circuit drops dramatically, thus pulmonary blood flow now goes into the lungs. The ductus arteriosus closes off.

But if the ductus remains open, then you have trouble. The blood flow goes from the high-pressure aorta through the ductus and into the pulmonary artery — a left-to-right shunt.

DUCTUS ARTERIOSUS

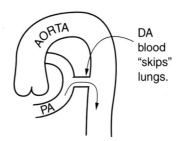

It would be cool to see the ductus itself on TEE, but that is hard to do. The ductus often falls into the "shadow" of the left mainstem bronchus, so you have to look for indirect signs:

- Chronic volume overload of the left atrium and ventricle.

- Left-to-right flow through the ductus itself (if you're lucky enough to see it).

- Diastolic ductal flow through the pulmonary artery.

- In the descending aorta, holodiastolic flow reversal (blood flows backward into the patent ductus). Of course, if the patient has aortic regurg, he or she would also have diastolic flow reversal. Can you have both at once (PDA and AR)? Sure.

So, overall, you have to see a constellation of things.

This could be a toughie on the test.

Coarctation of the Aorta

Reminder from the top of this section!

When you see one lesion, do a *complete* exam and look for *other* lesions. Coarctation of the aorta is the poster child for this idea, because coarctation of the aorta is associated with bicuspid aortic valve.

Just as the PDA can be hard to see, so also aortic coarctation can be hard to see, the lesion lying near the bothersome air-filled left mainstem bronchus. But, if you're lucky, you'll see this:

You can look for indirect signs:

- Highly pulsatile aortic root and akinetic abdominal aorta

- Rib notching on chest x-ray from enlarged intercostals trying to "find a way around the obstruction"

- Diminished lower extremity pulses (Imagine, you, a TEEologist, doing a physical exam. Incredible! Call *60 Minutes*, this is news!)

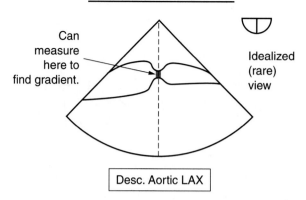

COARCTATION OF AORTA

Can measure here to find gradient.

Idealized (rare) view

Desc. Aortic LAX

On the test, you might get thrown because you might not see one of the "big 20," the TEE Alphabet views, but rather some angle you don't recognize. If you are *thinking* coarctation, you might tumble to the fact that there is a Doppler line in there, telling you they are measuring some flow somewhere in some occluded thing.

Aha! You'll say, they must be measuring a gradient across an occluded aorta. And there you have it.

Ebstein's Anomaly

After the toughies of the PDA and aortic coarctation (indirect signs, chest x-rays, physical exams — God Almighty, pretty soon you'll have to be a doctor again!), Ebstein's anomaly is a good old visual recognition thing that's easy to recognize.

Whew.

Take your normal four-chamber view and look at the tricuspid valves. Now move the leaflets deep into the ventricle. Voila!

EBSTEIN'S ANOMALY

Apical tricuspid valve

Atrialized right ventricle

ME 4-Chamber

Of note, the ventricle "above" the tricuspid valve often becomes "atri-alized," that is, becomes thin. The tricuspid valve itself doesn't work too well (no surprise), so you see tricuspid regurgitation.

Associated conditions? Wolff-Parkinson-White syndrome and right-to-left atrial shunts. That makes sense if you remember where the conduction system normally runs, then picture that same conduction system in the setting of an "atrialized" right ventricle.

Persistent Left Superior Vena Cava

You'll like this one because it's a rare chip shot.

Back to development-ville.

Vessels come and go, branchial clefts appear and disappear, all sorts of flippers and things arise out of the "ontogeny recapitulates phylogeny" soup and then go back into never-never land. If one of those "should go away" things sticks around, it turns into a question on the TEE exam, as well as a headache in the OR.

So it goes with the persistent left superior vena cava. You're *supposed* to have a *right* superior vena cava. If the *left* one sticks around, you get this left-sided (of the body) venous blood pouring into the coronary sinus (that's where the left superior vena cava ends). The coronary sinus then gets dilated.

Now the cool part. To peg this diagnosis, inject fluid into a left arm vein. The coronary sinus will light up like the 4th of July and pay off in silver dollars and you've got your diagnosis. Just how damned cool is that?

PERSISTENT LEFT SVC

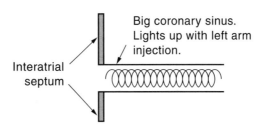

Big coronary sinus.
Lights up with left arm
injection.

Interatrial
septum

Tetralogy of Fallot

If you try to memorize all four things in the tetralogy of Fallot by rote, brutal memory, you might get tripped up. To make it happen, just draw a regular four-chamber view and move one little thing in the middle over a little bit. Gazingo, you've got it!

TETRALOGY OF FALLOT

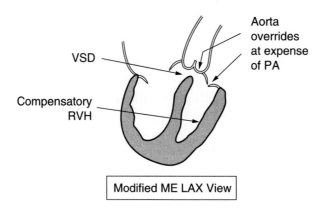

Modified ME LAX View

In words, here's what you're seeing, and then what you see on the TEE:

1. Overriding aorta

2. Pulmonic stenosis

3. VSD

4. RV hypertrophy (not so much part of the original problem as a "result" of the RV trying to push out the stenosed pulmonary outflow tract)

Transposition of the Great Arteries

Now the pictures start to get really weird, and you start crying out for pediatric cardiologists and such. Which baffle goes where is…well…uh…baffling to most of us mere mortals, but here's what it looks like and here's what the correction looks like:

TRANSPOSITION OF GREAT VESSELS

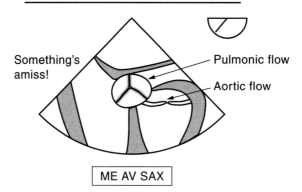

ME AV SAX

Some of the coolest echo images from the TEE meeting were adults coming back for follow-up after funky "switching" procedures as children. A point made at the meeting is this: thousands of people are living to adulthood who got these kiddy cardiac procedures. Try not to let your jaw drop too much when you see what looks like an alien life force in the middle of your patient's chest.

Atrioventricular Septal Defect — "AV Canal"

Look at the top half of a heart, with the atria amputated, to see the fibrous ring that holds the valves. This all has to come together just so. What can go wrong? You name it. Just fail to fuse here or there and a grab bag of defects can arise.

On echo, then, you can see any of an entire potpourri of pathology.

Conditions with Single Ventricular Physiology

A single ventricle will have to have some way of "sharing" the blood between systemic and pulmonary circulation, or else life itself would be impossible. (Sort of like "life without chemicals" in the old Dow Chemical TV commercials.)

Here's how single ventricles would look on echo:

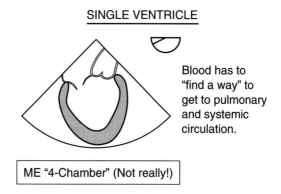

SINGLE VENTRICLE

Blood has to "find a way" to get to pulmonary and systemic circulation.

ME "4-Chamber" (Not really!)

XVII. Artifacts and Pitfalls

Imaging Artifacts

A must-see pair of lectures from the 2002 meeting is Dr. Heller's lecture on artifacts (perfectly illustrated with clear drawings and representative TEE images) and Dr. Grichnik's lecture on anatomic pitfalls (ditto on the drawings and representative TEEs). They are on the third tape, labeled #V01-02. If you can't afford the entire tape series, think seriously about just getting this one tape.

No can do? Then get the syllabus from the first half of the 2003 meeting. The pictures of the echo images don't reproduce well, but the explanations are excellent.

When you are in the OR, you are forever asking yourself, "Is it real, or is it Memorex?" We get seduced by the great images, and you have to shake yourself and say, "This is not a REAL LIVE picture, this is an ULTRASOUND CREATION OF A PICTURE, and ultrasound can fool you."

Let's grind through these monsters. Pay close, close, close attention to the aortic dissection artifacts; that is what will *scare hell* out of you in the middle of the night.

Useful for any and all artifacts is the mantra, "Change the viewing angle." That may allow you to see around a calcified or prosthetic valve. Plus, if you see the same thing from a bunch of different angles, guess what? It's really there! (Maybe. We live in an uncertain world.)

Shadowing   A strong reflector (e.g., metal valve or thick calcium) totally blocks the ultrasound wave and everything distal is eclipsed. As a matter of fact, that's what an eclipse is.

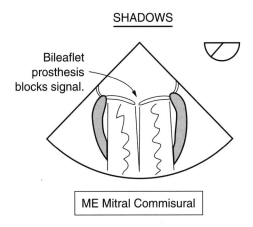

Reverberations   The beam bounces between a structure and a secondary reflector. Parallel lines go out from the object to the end of the image. The parallel lines follow the same path a shadow would, going from the point of bouncelage out to the end of the image.

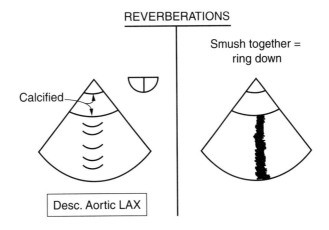

If these reverberations smush together, they appear as a solid line (a kind of "white shadow") that goes by the colorful moniker "ring down" or "comet tail," or "white shadow of reverberationess."

(I made that last one up.)

Refraction   Ultrasound gets bent from its original path and registers a structure in the wrong place, similar to seeing a straw "bend" as it goes into water. On TEE this is seen a lot in the descending aorta and gives rise to the appearance of a "double-barreled aorta."

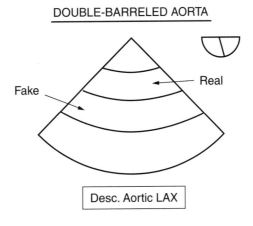

The mirror image is always on a straight line between the transducer and artifact and is always deeper than the true reflector.

You could see that double barrel and say, "Good golly, Miss Molly, we have a dissection!"

Side Lobes   Ultrasound sends out its major beam centrally, but side beams also come out. (You have to kind of look at this for a while before it sinks in. Side lobes generated some blank stares at the meeting.)

These side lobes can fake you out.

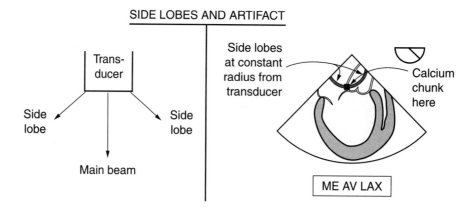

SIDE LOBES AND ARTIFACT

They hit a calcified thing, then "throw out" a shadow along a radial line from the calcified thing. Thus, the image will always look like a radius at a constant distance from the transducer.

Let the picture tell you what I'm stumbling to tell you.

Side lobes happen a lot in the real world.

Side lobes can look a LOT like a dissection.

Range Ambiguity At high pulse repetition frequency (don't be afraid to go back and look at the physics in Section V again), the ultrasound can get fooled into thinking an object is in the wrong location. A second pulse is sent out before the first one comes back, so the machine can't tell where the signal came from.

The end result of this chicanery? A Swan might appear in the left ventricle (oops!), or an aortic valve might appear in the middle of a chamber (how can the patient be so stable with his aortic valve sitting in the middle of the left ventricle?). Change the depth of the image (that will alter the pulse repetition frequency) and that should make the "mystery object" disappear.

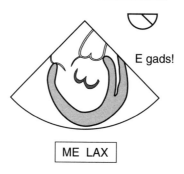

MISPLACED AORTIC VALVE

Resolution Headaches   Back to physics. The best resolution occurs at the focal zone of the beam. An object out of the focal zone will not appear clearly.

Enhancement   Not so tough. The flip side of shadowing. Instead of hitting a strong reflector, the beam hits a weak reflector; then the beam is attenuated less than normal, and the image appears brighter than usual. The usual example of this is seen in an image of the pericardium. Since it's hard to draw bright, I'll just label it as "bright."

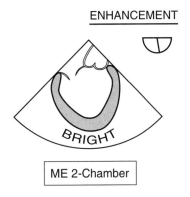

ENHANCEMENT

BRIGHT

ME 2-Chamber

Bovie Noise Surgeons   Humph. Can't live with 'em, can't gut them and hang them upside down outside the hospital; they'll write up an incident report on you and you'll be in committee hell for the rest of your life.

Bovie artifacts looks like a bunch of waves zapping around in your field. And it happens when you hear the Bovie go.

Doppler Artifacts and Pitfalls

The main Doppler headache, and a recurring point in the meeting and tapes, is aliasing. You will hear a million times (and no doubt be asked) to differentiate between continuous-wave Doppler (range ambiguity but no problem with aliasing) and pulsed-wave Doppler (range certainty but problems with aliasing).

As before, don't be afraid to go through the physics in Section V again. You finished physics a looooooooooooooooooooooong time ago, and this stuff can be a little tricky.

Aliasing   You can't measure a maximum velocity.

Wrong Angle   Remember the cosine thing from long ago in a galaxy far, far away? To get an accurate measure, you have to be looking "straight up the pipe."

If the angle is more than 20 degrees off kilter, your Doppler will be inaccurate.

Beam Width   This is the "Doppler equivalent" of the problem with side lobes. You are trying to see, for example, the left ventricular inflow from the left atrium, but your beam width is too wide and you also see an aortic regurgitant jet at the same time, screwing up the signal.

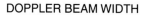
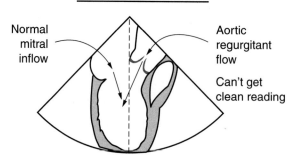

DOPPLER BEAM WIDTH

Normal mitral inflow

Aortic regurgitant flow

Can't get clean reading

Another problem with beam width is "the third dimension." The beams are not perfect 2-D structures. There is a thickness to them, so you may get an abnormal signal from something "out of the plane" of the image, but still "pick-upable" from the beam.

Mirror Image   Artifact A symmetric but weaker signal appears in the opposite direction of what you measure.

When this happens, reduce the gain.

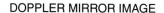
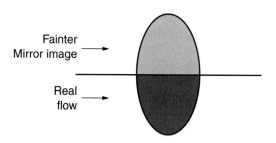

DOPPLER MIRROR IMAGE

Fainter Mirror image

Real flow

Ghosting   Remember the old chestnut about seeing the "green flash" of the sun *just* as it is setting? No doubt many a retina has gotten fried to a crisp looking for that. Ghosting is sort of like that.

With color Doppler, if the patient has a strong reflector like a metallic valve, you can get a brief flash of blue or red that doesn't correspond to any flow pattern. It's, like, you know man, just like this big flash, so don't get all bent out of shape, man.

Structures Mimicking Pathology

This is total Visual City, USA, and a lot of it you've heard of before.

All kinds of normal things and embryonic leftovers are floating around the heart, gumming up the works and throwing you for a loop. The list is quasi long, but each individual one just takes a little memory work and pattern recognition.

Moderator Band   A big muscle band in the apical third of the right ventricle (never in the left). The moderator band has part of the conduction system in it.

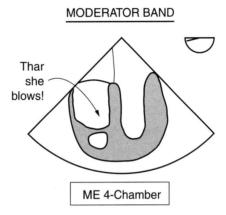

MODERATOR BAND

Thar she blows!

ME 4-Chamber

Pleural Effusion   Well, this isn't exactly *mimicking* pathology, hell, it IS pathology. But anyway, you see this lateral and posterior to the heart. Since the heart is on the left side (usually), you usually only see left pleural effusions.

Nodulus Arantii   Kick ass name, huh?

Little knobby fibrous thingies at the center of the free edge of each cusp of the aortic valve.

Dig the Latin name.

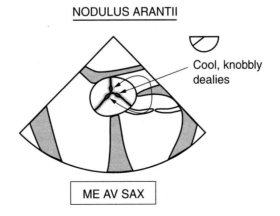

NODULUS ARANTII

Cool, knobbly dealies

ME AV SAX

Lambl's Excrescences Better name, even, than nodulus arantii. I hope I never get excrescences *anywhere*.

Filamentous thingamabobs attached (usually) to the aortic side of the aortic valve leaflets.

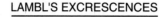

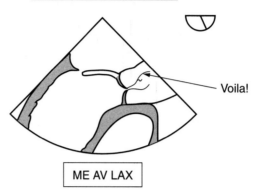

Coumadin Ridge Atrial tissue dividing the atrial appendage from the left upper pulmonary vein. Can look like a clot, but don't fall for it.

I already drew this once, don't get greedy.

Pectinate Muscles Parallel ridges along endocardial surfaces of the left and right atria, as well as both appendages.

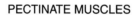

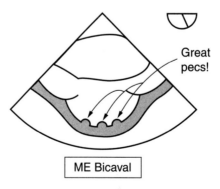

Crista Terminalis Little valve-like thingie at the junction of the superior vena cava and the right atrium (so you'll see it to the right side of a bi-caval view).

Eustachian Valve Same kind of deal over on the other side, where the inferior vena cava meets the right atrium.

Both of these were drawn a while ago.

Thebesian Valve   Same kind of deal, but now at the entrance to the coronary sinus. This can make it hard to place the retrograde cannula, since it is, in effect, a valve.

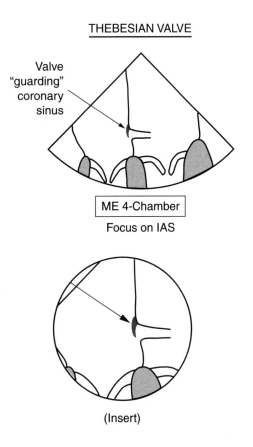

THEBESIAN VALVE

Valve "guarding" coronary sinus

ME 4-Chamber

Focus on IAS

(Insert)

Chiari Network   Kind of like a Lambl's excrescence in the atrium.

Wall Motion Abnormality   This isn't really an anatomic pitfall, but it's worth noting here, as Dr. Grichnik did in her lecture (and from which I hope she doesn't mind I stole everything!).

Epicardial pacing can make the septal wall appear hypokinetic or dyskinetic. The normal sequence of depolarization doesn't occur, so you could be fooled into thinking there was a coronary occlusion leading to this regional wall motion abnormality.

XVIII. Related Diagnostic Modalities

Stress Echocardiography

Stress echo with a TEE is the same deal as stress echo with a transthoracic echo (TTE). You get a baseline reading, then you crank the heart rate and contractility with a dobutamine infusion (5 to 20 micro-grams/kg/minute). What do you see?

- Normal myocardium: normal resting wall motion and hyper-dynamic function when you whip it with the dobutamine.

- At-risk myocardium: normal resting wall motion, then new wall motion abnormalities or worsening of systolic function with increasing dobutamine.

- Contractile reserve myocardium: baseline wall motion abnor-mality, but it improves with low-dose dobutamine. With this kind of myocardium, you might see a biphasic response, with worsening function at yet higher doses of dobutamine. You sort of shift into the "at-risk myocardium."

- Dead-as-a-doornail myocardium: nuthin', then more nuthin', then still later nuthin'.

Myocardial Perfusion Imaging

Instead of looking for wall motion abnormalities, there are new dyes that allow you to tag the blood and "see" the blood flow spreading out in the myocardium itself. The films of this are cosmic.

Epicardial Scanning

You can't do TEE on some people (those with esophageal pathology, 2% of "normal" people you can't get the probe in), so you go with epicardial scanning. Make sure the probe is covered with a sterile sheath (DUH) and has enough goop in the end of it so you can "stand off" a little and see well.

If the probe is jammed right smack dab up against something, you can't see it. Just like someone holding a piece of paper 1 mm from your eye.

When you see an epicardial image, you have to turn your brain upside down, because you are coming at things from a different direction.

As mentioned in the section on congenital anomalies, kiddie cardiac surgery often uses epicardial scanning. You're not hindered by bronchi getting in the way, so you can look all over the place.

Epi*aortic* scanning is the way to go for looking at aortic atherosclero-sis. People are trying to see if there is some goombah under the potential aortic cannulation site that will embolize and cause a stroke.

Contrast Echocardiography

Look at a regular TEE image. There is a lot of dropoff and uncertainty about the edges of the image, especially off to the sides.

With injectable echodense dye, the inside of the ventricle lights up and makes endocardial definition much easier.

This makes for more accurate estimation of cardiac outputs, plus lets you really see if a wall is moving or not (helpful for making wall motion abnormality calls).

Utility of TEE Relative to Other Diagnostic Modalities

You can look at this from a lot of different angles.

TEE Versus ECG

Regional wall motion abnormalities are the bomb when it comes to detecting ischemia.

First perfusion is disturbed, then diastolic dysfunction occurs (hard to pick up right away), then segmental wall motion abnormality occurs (TEE to the rescue!), then later ECG changes occur, and then later than that, chest pain occurs (unless, of course, the patient is denervated from diabetes or is post heart transplant).

So, to summarize, TEE is better than ECG to detect ischemia.

Of course, putting on an ECG ain't no biggie and placing a TEE is.

TEE Versus TTE (Transthoracic Echo)

Lot of pluses and minuses in this comparison.

TTE is easy to do in the awake patient and is comfortable. In the awake patient, TEE requires topicalization, sedation, and all the spooky aspects of a MAC anesthetic (oversedation, sympathetic stimulation — POP goes the aneurysm!)

TTE provides a better look at the front of the heart, though the ribs and lungs restrict your acoustic windows. The TEE provides a better look at the back of the heart, though there are some limitations to the windows here too.

With just the right window, TTE can get a look at the aortic arch that the TEE might miss. So in certain cases, TTE may be better at seeing a high arch dissection.

TEE Versus Coronary Angiography

Angiography wins the "visualize the coronaries" contest all hollow.

Femoral artery sticks are invasive, and can lead to pseudoaneurysms, retroperitoneal bleeds, and all kinda unholy terror. TEE obviates that, though TEE has its own complications.

TEE Versus Swan

TEE lets you see what's wrong in a hurry. A Swan may be hard to get in in a hurry (CVP is low, can't hit an IJ or a subclavian vein), and a Swan gives you numbers requiring some leap of faith. But a Swan "stays in" and may be useful for long-term ICU care. You can't be popping an echo every 5 minutes.

What's that up ahead, at the end of the yellow brick road? Is it the Emerald City?

No.

It looks like there is a problem.

3 · Hemodynamo-Doc

"Houston, we have a problem."

The crew of Apollo 13 solved their problems.

See if you can solve these.

The first time you see the quantitative problems of transesophageal echocardiography, you will defecate a quart jar of tenpenny nails, not to be too indelicate about it. But fear not, all is not lost. The math is no more complex than algebra, and the same concepts come back over and over and over again. The best way to show this is to plow through the problems they showed at the 2003 hemodynamics workshop meeting. The first time through (especially if you haven't seen this stuff before), it will seem like Greek. But by the end (once you see that the same equations reappear like Jason in a *Halloween* sequel), you should get it.

Go through these problems, and you, too, can be a Hemodynamo-Doc.

CASE 1   77-yo man having CABG surgery has an A-line, CVP, and (surprise) a TEE. On echo, the AV appears sclerosed with restricted leaflet motion and trace AR. His BSA is 2.0 meters squared. The following measurements are made:

- Heart rate: 75 bpm
- Systemic BP: 105/65 mm Hg
- CVP: 105/65 (Oops! The resident must have nailed big red! It's really 10 mm Hg.)
- Diameter LVOT: 2.2 cm
- TVI LVOT: 18 cm

- Peak velocity LVOT: 1.0 meters/second
- TVI AV: 62 cm
- Peak velocity AV: 3.4 meters/second
- Peak velocity TR: 2.8 m/sec

Your job, should you decide to accept it, is to calculate

- Stroke volume
- Cardiac output
- Cardiac index
- Peak right ventricular systolic pressure
- Peak aortic valve area
- Peak aortic valve gradient
- Peak left ventricular pressure

If you saw this problem ice cold, and thought the TEE exam was just a matter of looking at some videos and saying, "Yeah, there's a dissection," or "There's mitral regurg," then you would no doubt die right here and now. Fortunately, forewarned is forearmed; you KNOW this stuff will be on the test, so let's grind through it.

N. B.: There will be a LOT OF REPETITION here as we go through these problems. That is a good thing for it should POUND THIS STUFF THROUGH YOUR THICK SKULLS. At the echo course in San Diego, they emphasize that the course repeats and reinforces the main ideas.

Redundancy is a good thing.

And you can say that again.

Calculation of Stroke Volume

Volume of a cylinder = area of the cylinder × length of a cylinder

The stroke volume going through the heart is thought of as a "cylinder of blood," so you look for a place that has both an area that you can measure (lo and behold, the LVOT fits the bill) and a length that you can measure (the LVOT TVI, which is a "length"). TVI stands for *time-velocity integral*, and is measured by putting the pulsed-wave Doppler (the one that measures velocity at a *specific place*) right in the LVOT. Then you trace the outside of the velocity curve. The computer in the

TEE machine will give you a time-velocity integral, which is, the length that the blood moved.

There is a little leap of faith here, with only engineers and pencil-necked geeks understanding exactly the nature of "integration" turning a velocity in cm/second into a length of cm. Suffice it to say, TVI gives you the length that the cylinder of blood moved.

> Volume of a cylinder of blood moving through the heart (which is the stroke volume) = area at a specific place (here, the LVOT) × length at a specific place (here, the TVI of the LVOT)

Cleaning up a little,

> Stroke volume = area LVOT × TVI LVOT

Area of a circle, you recall from 8th grade or so, is pi × radius squared. Since pi is 3.14 and since radius = diameter divided by 2, then the area equation can be simplified to area = 3.14 × diameter squared/2 squared, or 3.14 × diameter squared/4. Crank out a little division and you come up with

> Area = 0.785 × diameter squared

For some reason, in the TEE review course, they always go with area = 0.785 × diameter squared, they never go with pi × radius squared. Whatever, when in Rome, do as the Romans.

So let's wander back to the stroke volume thing.

> Stroke volume = area LVOT × TVI LVOT
>
> = 0.785 × (2.2 cm) squared × 18 cm
>
> = 3.8 cm squared × 18 cm
>
> = 68 cm cubed, or 68 ml

As you do these problems, pay attention to two things:
1. Units
2. Common sense

The units should come out properly, just like in chemistry or physics class. We ended up with a stroke volume in units of cm cubed, or in other words, ml. That makes sense. That is how you usually measure stroke volume. If, after your crafty machinations, you had come up with units of, say, hectares per nanosecond per light-year, then you must ask yourself, "When was the last time I measured a stroke volume in hectares per nanosecond per light-year?" The answer being, "Never," you should go back and redo the math.

Common sense should also play a part in your answer. This patient, ailing though he was, had a stroke volume of 68 ml. That is not the greatest, but is compatible with life in a human being. If, in blazing contrast, your calculated stroke volume came out to 3 ml, then you would have to ask yourself, "Just how long does your average human being live with a stroke volume of 3 ml?"

I wouldn't sell such a person life insurance.

The flip side of the coin is, what if you calculate a stroke volume of 8900 ml? Either you are calculating the stroke volume of King Kong, or you made a decimal point mistake in there somewhere.

Do your problem, then step back. Look at the units. Use common sense.

Calculation of Cardiac Output

Oh happiness, you don't need any TEE chicanery to generate this number. This is just plain old anesthesia knowledge stuff.

Cardiac output = stroke volume × heart rate

= 68 ml/heart beat × 75 heart beats/minute

= 5.1 L/minute

Does it pass the "units make sense" test? Yes. Does it pass the "common sense" test? Yes. You're in business.

Calculation of Cardiac Index

Would that it were all this easy! This goes back to Anesthesia 101.

Cardiac index = cardiac output/surface area

= 5.1 L/minute divided by 2 meters squared

= 2.5 L/minute/meter squared

Calculation of Peak Right Ventricular Systolic Pressure

Sorry, the free ride is over, you'll have to put your thinking cap back on for this one.

For this, you'll need two things, one mathematical, and one commonsensical/visual.

The Mathematical

The Bernoulli equation will appear a million times in any discussion of TEE. The complicated form of this equation takes Sir Isaac Newton to decipher, but the simplified version comes to us as the digestible

> Delta P (the change in pressure between two chambers in a flowing system) = 4 × velocity squared (where the velocity is measured at a "choke point" or narrowing between the two chambers)

So picture the place we're interested in measuring, here the right ventricle. Where is there a "choke point" or narrowing that leads into or out of the right ventricle, we can measure a velocity. (Remember, the TEE can measure a *velocity* for you, but it cannot measure a *pressure*.)

Aha! The patient has tricuspid regurgitation, and there is a measurement of the tricuspid regurg velocity that we can measure:

> Peak velocity TR = 2.8 meters/second

(Note well, the units for the Bernoulli equation work out as follows — use the velocity in meters/second and your gradient will come out in mm Hg.)

So let's convert that TR velocity into a gradient:

> Delta P (in mm Hg) = 4 × velocity (in meters/second) squared
>
> = 4 × (2.8 meters/second) squared
>
> = 31 mm Hg

Now on to the second thing you need to solve this problem.

The Commonsensical/Visual

So we want to know the pressure in one place, we have a gradient, and we have a pressure in a second place. Here's where the common sense comes in.

There is a higher pressure place, the right ventricle (that's what contracts, after all). There is a lower pressure place, the atrium (the pressure in that thin-walled chamber better be lower than the thicker walled ventricle).

Common sense tells you that you could set up an equation like this:

The higher pressure place – the gradient you lose as you go to the lower pressure place = the pressure you have left over in the lower pressure place

The right ventricle – the gradient going back into the atrium = the pressure in the atrium

Unknown – 31 mm Hg you lose going across the tricuspid valve = 10 mm Hg (the CVP, or, the pressure in the right atrium)

Unknown – 31 mm Hg = 10 mm Hg

Unknown = 41 mm Hg

In the TEE review course, they said

Right ventricular systolic pressure = CVP + gradient

This may work for you, but I found it more useful to think through the problem from the vantage of "here's the high-pressure area, here's the low-pressure area, and here's the loss of pressure between them." That way you'll understand the way the pressure works, and you'll be less likely to, say, subtract the CVP from the gradient rather than add the CVP to the gradient. Once you're done, you can then draw your picture and see if common sense holds up.

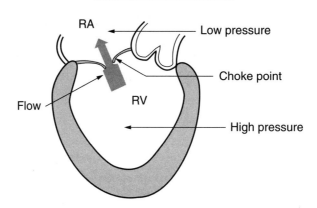

MAPPING PRESSURES

Calculation of Peak Aortic Valve Area

Here the continuity equation comes home to roost. At first baffling, the continuity equation makes sense; it's just a question of cross multiplying and dividing, and shouldn't make you lose much sleep.

Why bother? Why not just draw a line around the open aortic valve and let the TEE machine do the area for you by planimetry?

Ah, grasshopper, things are not so simple as they seem.

Planimetry, as so many things in life, only works when you *don't need it*! (Kind of like the umbrella that never leaks unless it rains, or the life preserver that doesn't let you drown unless you happen to fall into the ocean.) When the aortic valve is crunchy and stenotic, planimetry (a two-dimensional exercise), just cannot get a good handle on the exact orifice area. You outline up here, but there is more stenosis below your outline, or there is more stenosis above your planimetry, so the planimetry is just no good.

> Continuity Equation Idea: Flow through one area of the heart equals flow through another area of the heart.

Fluids are not compressible, so you can't "squish" the blood. Also, blood cannot just "disappear," which brings up the BIG EXCEPTION to the continuity equation:

> If a patient has noncontinuous flow (septal defect somewhere), then you can't use the continuity equation. To use continuity, have continuity!

So, if you can measure flow through one area, then that should equal flow in another area.

Flow here = flow there. The essence of the continuity equation.

Recall from earlier that we "create" measurable flow by assuming a cylindrical amount of blood flow. (We did that in the original part of this problem, the stroke volume problem. Go back now and nail that down, because that is the heart of the continuity equation.) We measure this cylindrical flow by getting one area and multiplying it by the length (the time-velocity integral), thus getting flow.

> Area × length = area × length

We know we want to know the aortic valve area, so where can we find another place to measure stuff?

The left ventricular outflow tract, of course! (The LVOT is forever bailing our mathematical asses out of trouble.)

So flow through the LVOT should equal flow through the aortic valve. So plug in the respective three things that we DO have, and solve for the one thing we don't have:

> Area of the LVOT blood flow "cylinder" × length that the blood flow "cylinder" goes = area of the aortic valve "cylinder" × length that the aortic blood flow "cylinder" goes

> Area LVOT × TVI LVOT = *unknown* aortic valve area × TVI aortic valve

You have the diameter of the LVOT, 2.2 cm, so use the area formula:

> Area = pi × radius squared, *or,*

> Area = 0.785 × diameter squared

> = 0.785 × (2.2 cm) squared

> = 3.8 cm squared

So, plodding along,

> 3.8 cm squared (the area of the LVOT) × 18 cm (TVI of the LVOT) = *unknown* (the area of the aortic valve) × 62 cm (the TVI of the AV)

Cross multiply and divide, solving for the area of the aortic valve, and, voila!

> Area of the aortic valve = 1.1 cm squared

Does this pass the units test? Yes. Aortic valve areas are measured in cm squared.

Does this pass the common sense test? Yes, this fits the general size you would expect of a stenotic aortic valve. You didn't get an aortic valve area the size of an electron, nor did you get an area the size of Comiskey Park.

Now hold on to your slide rulers and cyclotrons — there is, it turns out, another way to get the aortic valve area.

Go back to the cylinder of blood idea (the gist of all these equations). If you look just at the aortic valve, you could say:

Aortic valve area × TVI aortic valve = stroke volume through the aortic valve

So, if you were of a mind to, you could calculate the aortic valve area that way, could you not? (The first time you see this, you'll go, "Huh? Aren't they cheating?") But it's actually not cheating, because, in order to get the stroke volume, you had to use the concept of the "cylinder of blood going through the LVOT" (see above, where we calculated the very first part of this problem, the stroke volume).

Take a second to digest this.

No, really, look back up there, don't take this on faith.

Satisfied? Good.

So, here we go with the second way to calculate the area of the aortic valve.

Area of the aortic valve × TVI of the aortic valve = stroke volume
Unknown (area of the aortic valve) × 62 cm = 68 cm cubed

Cross multiply and divide, and gee whiz golly, the aortic valve area is *still* 1.1 cm squared.

That shouldn't surprise you, as this patient hasn't aged much during this problem.

What *should* surprise you is a second answer *different* from your first. Since you were just grinding the same numbers through in different ways, you *should* get a second answer the same as the first. If you don't, go back and rework it.

Calculation of Peak Aortic Valve Gradient

A little less Sturm und Drang here. Just use the Bernoulli equation:

Delta P (the pressure gradient across a "choke point" in a flowing system) = 4 × velocity in the "choke point" squared
Delta P = 4 × (3.4 meters/second) squared

(Keep in mind, you need that velocity in meters/second to get a pressure in mm Hg!)

Delta P = 46 mm Hg

Units OK? Check.

Common sense OK? Check.

Calculation of Peak Left Ventricular Pressure

At the TEE course, they didn't ask for this, but it's worth doing just to get that "high-pressure area, gradient loss, low-pressure area" idea down.

First, draw a picture of what you're trying to find. (To repeat, getting the concept down of where the high pressure should be, as well as where the low pressure should be, is important. A good picture will make sure you add where you should add and subtract where you should subtract.)

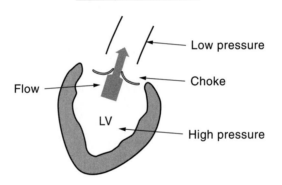

The high-pressure area should be the left ventricle in systole, because the left ventricle has to overcome the "choke point" of the aortic valve, and still have enough oomph left over to provide systolic pressure.

High pressure in the left ventricle (unknown) – pressure lost in the stenotic aortic valve (the previously calculated gradient of 46 mm Hg) = pressure left over in the aorta (the systolic pressure of 105 mm Hg)

Unknown – 46 mm Hg = 105 mm Hg

Unknown = 151 mm Hg

Now, redraw the picture and see if it makes sense.

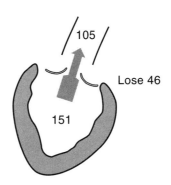

CASE 2   48-yo man having CABG. Monitoring includes a finger on the pulse and an anesthesiologist on the phone to Merrill-Lynch. OK, OK, sorry. Monitoring includes an A-line, CVP, and TEE. LV appears dilated and hypocontractile. There is a central jet of MR judged to be 2+ to 3+ in severity. The following measurements are made:

- Diameter LVOT: 2.5 cm

- TVI LVOT: 13 cm

- Mitral annular diameter: 3.5 cm

- TVI mitral annular diameter: 11 cm

- PISA radius: 0.8 cm

- PISA alias velocity: 34 cm/second

- Peak velocity MR: 574 cm/second

- TVI MR: 172 cm

Calculate the following:

- LVOT stroke volume

- MV stroke volume

- MV regurgitant volume

- MV regurgitant fraction

- Regurgitant orifice area

- PISA calculations

    Regurgitant flow rate

    Regurgitant orifice area

    Regurgitant volume

    Regurgitant fraction

Before you regurgitate yourself at all this stuff, a few pointers.

On this, the math part of the test, they will just give you the various measures. They'll lay LVOT diameter on a silver platter and hand it to you. In other parts of the test, you will visually have to show exactly where you would take this measurement yourself. And on the test the various places are damned close to one another, so make sure you know where to take these measurements.

Second, PISA makes the whole auditorium groan, it seems so esoteric at first. But once you gird your loins and throw yourself into this stuff, you'll see that PISA is just the continuity equation in another form.

Flow through the PISA = flow through another area

PISA's area is a hemisphere, so that's a little different.

PISA's area is affected by its angle to the valve, so that's a little different.

PISA implies you know what the hell aliasing is, so that's a little different.

Alright, so PISA is a pain in the ass, what can I tell you? I didn't make up the exam!

Let's take a little breather from the PISA monster, get as far along as we can in the calculations, get a little confidence, then jump into the snake pit of PISA-ness.

Calculation of LVOT Stroke Volume

Whew, this is review. If you got the karma of the first case, this should be cake. I'll go through it just as slowly, though, so we jam this stuff into your sulci but good.

From the chaos and irregularity of a real-live stroke volume, we make up a "pretend" stroke volume that magically looks like a perfect cylinder, with a perfect area and length.

Next, we look at the LVOT, make our area calculation, then multiply it by the length (the TVI):

Stroke volume LVOT = area LVOT × length LVOT

Stroke volume = pi × radius square × TVI

Or, in TEE Course-speak:

Stroke volume = 0.785 × diameter squared × TVI

$$= 0.785 \times (2.5 \text{ cm}) \text{ squared} \times 13 \text{ cm}$$

$$= 64 \text{ cm cubed, or } 64 \text{ ml}$$

Units make sense? Yes. Common sense rule checks out? Yes. (Make it a habit to always do this two-part checkout.)

Calculation of MV Stroke Volume

Danger! Danger, Will Robinson! Remember, when you measure these, to measure both the diameter and the TVI *at the same place*. In this problem, be sure to measure both the diameter of the mitral valve and the TVI of the mitral valve at the *annulus*. If you measure the diameter at the annulus and the TVI at, say, the tips of the mitral valve, then you would get an inaccurate result.

Stroke volume of mitral valve = area of mitral valve × length of flow in mitral valve (the TVI)

So once again, we are invoking a "cylinder of blood flow."

Though the mitral valve is more like an oval, for purposes of this problem, we will consider it a circle:

Stroke volume = pi × radius squared × TVI

Or, bowing to TEE convention:

Stroke volume = 0.785 × diameter squared × TVI

$$= 0.785 \times (3.5 \text{ cm}) \text{ squared} \times 11 \text{ cm}$$

$$= 106 \text{ cm cubed, or } 106 \text{ ml}$$

Units check? Yes. Common sense check? Wait a minute! Didn't we just calculate an LVOT stroke volume of 64 ml? Now where did this stroke volume of 106 ml come from? What about the Holiest of Holies, the continuity equation?

Confused? Pause for a moment and think about what's happening.

This patient has mitral regurgitation, so it makes sense that *more* should go through the mitral valve than goes out the LVOT. Some of that mitral volume is lost by going backward (as we'll see below). Recall, too, that the continuity equation doesn't apply here, because the LVOT measurement applies to blood flowing out to the aorta during *systole*. The blood flow going forward through the mitral valve occurs during *diastole*.

Systole and diastole do not occur at the same time. They are *DIS*continuous so the continuity equation does *not* apply to them.

So, in review, the units check and the common sense also checks, once you think about what is happening and *when* it is happening.

Calculation of MV Regurgitant Volume

Now it starts to come together.

> Regurgitant volume through the mitral valve = total volume that goes through the mitral valve – total volume that goes out through the aortic valve

Another warning for Will Robinson.

This calculation only holds if there is no aortic regurgitation as well. The extra flow that comes back during aortic regurgitation would mix in with the blood regurgitating through the mitral valve, and all bets are off on volume calculations.

Adding aortic regurg to mitral regurg takes you from one equation–one unknown to one equation–two unknowns, and that is a no-no.

> Regurg volume = 106 ml – 64 ml

> = 42 ml

Units check? Yes. Common sense check? Ye-e-e-es. (If you find yourself hesitating, draw a picture to satisfy yourself that it does, indeed, make sense.)

Calculation of MV Regurgitant Fraction

No rocket science here.

> Regurgitant fraction of mitral valve = regurgitant volume
> MV/total volume through MV

> = 42 ml/106 ml

> = 0.4

or, in percentage terms, regurgitant percentage = 40%.

Units check? Yes, there are no units.

Common sense check? Yes, you can see a regurgitant valve tossing 40% backward. That goes along with significant regurg.

You'll note you didn't come up with something impossible, like a regurgitant percentage of 178% or a regurgitant percentage of –5%. Thank heaven for small miracles.

Calculation of Regurgitant Orifice Area

This is a little hypothetical, as the regurgitant orifice area is not a fixed thing that instantly appears, then instantly disappears. In reality, it's more like a door that is closed, opens at a certain speed, stays open for a length of time, and then closes at a certain speed. This calculation looks at the "door all the way open" and ignores the reality of the "opening period" and the "closing period."

But you're not here to think. Just do the calculation and keep your trap shut.

Go back to our cylinder of blood and start calculating.

Regurgitant orifice area × length (the TVI of regurgitation) = stroke volume of regurgitation

Regurgitant orifice area × 172 cm = 42 cm cubed

Cross multiply and divide, you busy little hemodynamic beavers.

Regurgitant orifice area = 0.24 cm squared

Units check? Yep. Common sense check? U-u-uh.

That makes sense. The mitral valve isn't a *complete* waste case; it is regurgitant, but not wide, wide open, so it makes sense that a portion, not all, of the valve effectively "stays open" during systole, allowing for the 40% regurgitation.

PISA Calculations

Hunker down, cowboys and cowgirls, it's not so bad as you think. Before we go into the actual calculations in this case, let's go over the main aspects of PISAtology.

Look at the words that make up PISA, and draw pictures to illustrate the point.

Proximal That means the colorful and troublesome PISA radius will appear on the upstream part of the "choke point." So draw a few pictures. If the patient has mitral regurg, and the flow is pouring from the high-pressure left ventricle into the low-pressure left atrium, the PISA will appear where?

Proximal! That is, the PISA will appear in the left ventricle, the "near" side of the "choke point." The proximal area of the choke hold, not the far side. That would be "*distal* isovelocity surface area," and if you think of the chaotic flow on the far side of a "choke point," that doesn't make sense.

How about a case of mitral stenosis? Flow is trying to "squeeze" through a tight mitral valve. Where would the PISA radius appear then?

Proximal! On the near side of the choke point, that is, in the left atrium.

Again, a radius on the *far* side of the choke point doesn't make sense.

Isovelocity All the flow at that area is the same. Recall that flow Doppler is a *pulsed-wave*, not a continuous-wave, phenomenon. At a certain velocity, the color of the wave will change. Conveniently for us, the aliasing velocity (the velocity where color change occurs) is listed on the machine.

Well, why should the isovelocity thing line up so perfectly for us. Why isn't the isovelocity thing scattered all over the map?

Think of water going toward a narrow sluice gate. The velocities are all over the map, until you get real close; then the pressure bearing down on the water is all the same. The velocities "organize" as the water gets closer to the sluice gate, and you get a hemisphere of water all going the same speed toward that narrow opening. That is why you get a hemisphere of "isovelocity-ness" that appears on the TEE screen.

Surface Area Unlike earlier equations, which used the area of a circle (pi × radius squared), this area is that of a hemisphere (2 × pi × radius squared). Why? Look at the PISA thing. It is a hemisphere, not a circle.

So that's where you get the 2 × pi × radius squared. In calculations done at the conference, they give you the radius and you go with 6.28 (that is, 2 × 3.14) × radius squared.

So once you believe in PISA, have the formula for area of a hemisphere down, and recall the continuity equation, you are in business.

Calculation of Regurgitant Flow Rate by PISA

Just as in other valve calculations, invent the idea of a cylinder of blood flowing along with a certain area and a certain length. This requires a little mind bending, as you are used to looking at the area of a circle and multiplying it by the length. Here, with PISA calling the shots, you make an *area of a hemisphere* and multiply it by the length.

Try not to think about it too much, you might pop an aneurysm. Just go with the flow.

Regurgitant flow rate = PISA area × aliasing velocity

Wait, wait! Where did that aliasing velocity come from again?

That line, where the flow changes color, must all be going at the same velocity — remember the water flowing towards the sluice gate? So read the aliasing velocity right off your TEE screen (it's listed right next to a colored bar), measure the radius to that line change, and you know that *right there*, the blood has to be going *that fast*, the aliasing velocity. And you measured the radius right there, where the color change occurs, so you are satisfying the demand that the area and the velocity be measured at the same place. So,

Area (in one specific place) × velocity (at that same specific place) = volume (at that specific place)

Regurgitant flow rate = 2 × pi × (0.8 cm) squared × 34 cm/second

Wait, wait! In all the other stuff, we used TVI and got a length in cm. Now we've got this aliasing velocity that has cm/second. Doesn't that screw everything up?

Don't panic. Take a deep breath. The question asked for a regurgitant flow rate (which implies a flow per unit time), so the aliasing velocity–is-not-the-same-as-TVI will not screw us up. But it's good to see you fretting about the units.

Regurgitant flow rate = 6.28 × (0.8 cm) squared × 34 cm/second

= 137 cm cubed/second

Units OK? Check. (Again, you get Brownie points if you got nervous about the aliasing velocity not being the same as the TVI). Common sense? Yes.

Calculation of Regurgitant Orifice Area by PISA

Here we'll keep an especially close eye on the units.

As before, area times velocity will equal flow. (Remember how we did the same thing with other valves and other flows. It always goes back to the same thing: area × velocity = flow. In earlier calculations, we didn't have the confounding variable of aliasing velocity, with its pesky cm/second. Before, we always had a TVI with just cm. Watch closely.)

> Effective regurgitant orifice area (of regurgitant mitral valve) × velocity (through the mitral valve [recall, we can measure velocities directly, but not pressures]) = flow (through mitral valve)

In shorter form,

> ERO × velocity MR peak = flow (calculated by PISA)

Note, the velocity MR peak is in cm/second, and our flow by PISA is in cm cubed/second, so that pesky second will cancel out:

> ERO × 574 cm/second = 137 cm cubed/second

Cross multiply and divide and you get ERO = 0.24 cm squared.

Units OK? Yes. Common sense OK? Well now, I will be dipped in hot fudge, stuck on a stick, and served up at the County Fair — the ERO turned out to be the same thing! 0.24 cm squared. And this time we really *did* calculate it a different way.

Who'd a thunk it.

Damnation.

Calculation of Regurgitant Volume by PISA

Area × length, area × length, area × length. Do you see a pattern here?

> Regurgitant volume = effective regurgitant area × TVI of the regurgitant valve

= 0.24 cm squared (what we just calculated) × 172 cm

= 41 cm cubed

Units? Check. Common sense? Check. Recall, with the other way, we calculated a regurgitant volume of 42 ml. That is close enough for government work.

Calculation of Regurgitant Fraction by PISA

Well, after jumping through all those other flaming hoops, this is nothin' but nothin'.

Regurgitant fraction (PISA method) = 41 cm cubed/ 106 cm cubed

= 0.39

or, in percentage terms, 39%, which makes both units and common sense sense. (Or, [sense] squared.)

Now that problem right there is a killer. If you can smack through that, you can handle most anything in the hemodynamic front. Might be worth going over this again a couple times, making sure you keep getting the units all squared away, especially with PISA's little twists and turns.

CASE 3   60-yo obese female s/p cardiac arrest following total hip replacement. Patient is brought to the operating room based upon a preliminary TEE that suggests pulmonary embolus.

> **CONFERENCE NOTE**   There was an entire lecture on TEE in the evaluation of hypoxemia, and it focused on how TEEs help diagnose pulmonary emboli. Though the embolus itself is rarely seen, the secondary signs — RV dilatation, tricuspid regurg, all the signs of a right heart struggling to push blood past an obstruction — are most helpful in making this slippery diagnosis of pulmonary embolus.

They did show one unbelievable clip of an enormous embolus that actually was in transit through the right heart. On screen, in real time, it came unglued, shot up into the pulmonary artery, and the patient went on to die soon after. Scary as hell. About as impressive a TEE as you'd ever care to see. Or not see.

VITAL SIGNS

- Heart rate: 100 bpm

- Systemic BP: 110/60 mm Hg

- CVP: 16 mm Hg

TEE DATA

- Pulmonary artery diameter: 2.0 cm

- Pulmonary artery TVI: 10 cm

- Aortic valve TVI: 15 cm

- TR peak velocity: 4 meters/second

CALCULATE

- Stroke volume

- Cardiac output

- Peak right ventricular systolic pressure

- Aortic valve area

You've done two of these already, and you should have the equipment to figure these out on your own, so give it a try before you read on. You will note that the same stuff keeps coming up, the same ideas, the same equations. But it still doesn't hurt to draw a picture or two to keep the big picture in mind.

This is a heart whose right side is "stopped up" with a plug in the outflow from the right ventricle to the lungs. *Status hemicardioconstipationatus dextrus*, if you prefer the Latin term. The tricuspid regurg shouldn't surprise you. As the right ventricle groans against a high pressure, some blood will go backward through the tricuspid valves.

Calculation of Stroke Volume

Find an area, find a TVI, and create your cylinder of blood flow to give you your volume. No problem, we've done it before.

OK, roll up the sleeves, find that LVOT diameter, find that LVOT TVI, and plug them into the equation:

Flow = area × length

So, flow = 0.785 × (diameter of LVOT) squared × TVI of the LVOT

SCREEEEEEEEEEEEEEEEEEEEEEEEEEEEEEEEEEEEEECH!

What the hell? Where are my old favorites? How can this be? Has the world turned upside down? It was so EASY to see it that way. You're looking right down the pipe of the left ventricular escape hatch. Out goes the blood through the LVOT into the aorta and you're there! What am I supposed to do with the information I *do* have?

Here's where you really need to *understand* the continuity equation. The information you get is the pulmonary artery diameter and the pulmonary artery TVI. If you really believe, I mean believe, brothers and sisters, in the sanctity of the continuity equation, then you must convince yourself that flow through the pulmonary artery will equal flow through the aorta.

That is, if the forward flow has no weird places the blood could disappear to (ventricular septal defect, atrial septal defect, some weird AV malformation in the lung).

But! But! What about the tricuspid regurg? Doesn't that "undo" the continuity equation?

No. The TVI you measure through the pulmonary artery is real-live, forward flow. That flow has made it *past* the right ventricle. Whatever went backward went backward, and we'll measure that in our own sweet time. But the TVI of the forward flow through the PA will rock right on straight through to the lungs, the left atrium, and the left ventricle, and out into the body.

> **If no flow goes backward from the pulmonary artery on out (that is, the pulmonary artery itself is not regurgitant), then the continuity equation says, "the flow will flow."**

So, now that we've settled that, then we can calculate our stroke volume:

Stroke volume = area of the PA × TVI of the PA, *or,*

Stroke volume = 0.785 × diameter squared × TVI

$$= 0.785 \times (2 \text{ cm}) \text{ squared} \times 10 \text{ cm}$$

$$= 31 \text{ cm cubed, or } 31 \text{ ml}$$

Units check? Yes. Common sense check? That forward flow seems pretty small. In earlier patients we were getting stroke volumes of 68 ml and the like. Only 31 ml? Pretty punky. But then, what does common sense tell you? This patient has a big PE, a big blockage to flow out of her right ventricle. It's conceivable and understandable that a monster plug to the RV could cut the "usual" stroke volume in half. So, yes, this passes the common sense test.

While you're at it, turn the logic around. What if you calculate a stroke volume greater than normal, say, 90 ml? That wouldn't jibe with the picture of a pulmonary embolus and blocked forward flow.

Always check your numbers against common sense and what is really happening to the patient. You will be less likely to make a mistake. If you just plug in numbers and hope against hope that you're right, you'll stumble.

Calculation of Cardiac Output

Cardiac output is stroke volume × heart rate. Go back to your belief in the continuity equation — the flow we measure going through the pulmonary artery IF FLOW CONTINUES STRAIGHT THROUGH WITHOUT MITRAL REGURG, AORTIC REGURG, OR SOME SEPTAL DEFECT should be the flow going through the aorta.

$$\text{Cardiac output} = 31 \text{ cm cubed /heart beat} \times 100 \text{ heart beats/minute}$$

$$= 3.1 \text{ L/minute}$$

Calculation of Peak Right Ventricular Systolic Pressure

Here again a picture will keep your signs straight. Whether on the right side or the left side of the heart, think of what's going on (here, systolic flow from the right ventricle into the right atrium through the "choke point" of the regurgitant tricuspid valve), think of where the highest pressure should be (here, the right ventricle), the place where the gradient will occur (the tricuspid valve), and the low-pressure place (the right atrium). So, the equation will say

Right ventricle (a high-pressure unknown) – gradient at the choke point (the tricuspid valve) = pressure in the low-pressure place (the right atrium)

How to measure the "choke point"? We have a velocity (which TEE can measure). Plug in Bernoulli:

Delta P = 4 × velocity squared

Delta P = 4 × (4 meters/second) squared (Remember, velocity in meters/second to get pressure in mm Hg.)

Delta P = 64 mm Hg

Right ventricle peak pressure − pressure gradient = low-pressure atrium pressure

RV peak pressure − 64 mm Hg = 16 mm Hg

RV peak pressure = 80 mm Hg

Units check? Yes. Common sense? Yes.

Now, apply your common sense to the clinical scene. Here's a patient with a PE big enough to give her cardiac arrest. She has little forward flow (bad stroke volume, bad cardiac output). Her right ventricle, which in a normal patient generates peak pressures of, say 25 or 30 mm Hg, is now generating a whopping 80 mm Hg. And with that high a right ventricular pressure, is it any wonder that the tricuspid valve (with a whiff of regurg in the best of times) is pouring blood backward?

It all fits. The numbers match the clinical reality. Isn't science wonderful?

Calculation of Aortic Valve Area

Back to the continuity equation (didn't I tell you you just keep doing the same stuff over and over again?).

In days of yore, we did this with the LVOT, remember?

Area LVOT × TVI LVOT = area AV (the *unknown*) × TVI AV

Then you just cross multiply and divide. Well, as noted above, we ain't got no LVOT. We got the PA. There is tricuspid regurg, but that doesn't concern us now. We're past that level of the regurg, and if, from the PA forward, there is no stop to forward, continuous flow, we should be able to use the continuity equation.

Plug in:

Area PA × TVI PA = area AV (the *unknown*) × TVI AV

0.785 × (2.0 cm) squared × 10 cm = area AV × 15 cm

Cross multiply and divide, you get AV area = 2 cm squared.

Units check? Yes. Areas are in cm squared. Common sense check? Yes, 2 cm squared puts this woman's aortic valve area in the normal range. And nowhere was there mention of aortic stenosis. She's got enough trouble already, what with a PE and cardiac arrest. Let's not give her more worries.

Go back to Case 1. Remember how we worked out the AV area another way?

Aortic valve area × TVI AV = stroke volume

We can do that here, also:

Aortic valve area × 15 cm = 31 cm cubed

= 2 cm squared

As before, this shouldn't come across as some miracle, as you are just regrinding the numbers in a different path to get to the same result. Of course, if you regrind and come out with a different number, perhaps you need to look things over and mend the error of your ways.

CASE 4 60-yo male with acute aortic dissection and aortic insufficiency.

VITAL SIGNS

- Heart rate: 80 bpm
- Systemic BP: 120/60 mm Hg

TEE DATA

- LVOT diameter: 2.0 cm
- LVOT TVI: 30 cm
- MV diameter: 3 cm
- MV TVI: 10 cm
- AI TVI: 160 cm
- AI end-diastolic velocity: 3 meters/second

CALCULATE

- LVOT stroke volume
- Mitral valve stroke volume

- Aortic regurgitant volume

- Aortic regurgitant fraction

- Aortic regurgitant orifice area

- Cardiac output

- Left ventricular end-diastolic pressure

Calculation of LVOT Stroke Volume

Some things never change, ain't it grand.

Make your cylinder of blood flow. Get the area of the LVOT – pi × radius squared, or, 0.785 × diameter squared. Then get your length of your cylinder of blood, the TVI – 30 cm.

LVOT stroke volume = 0.785 × (2.0 cm) squared × 30 cm

= 94 cm cubed

It's worth reminding yourself *where* you get all these numbers from. You measure the LVOT about 5 to 10 mm proximal to the annulus of the aortic valve. You measure the LVOT velocity (around which you draw your cursor to get the TVI) at the EXACT SAME PLACE, using… well, you tell me. Do you use continuous-wave Doppler or pulsed-wave Doppler?

(Play the theme from Jeopardy here.)

Right, pulsed-wave Doppler. Pulsed wave gives you a *specific* velocity at a *specific* place, unlike continuous wave, which gives you ALL velocities along a line. (If this is still a mystery to you, review the difference between continuous wave and pulsed wave in Chapter 2; you need to know this ice cold.)

Calculation of Mitral Valve Stroke Volume

Same deal here. Create your cylinder of blood, get an area, get a length, and you're in business. Again, we'll "round out" the "what is really oval" mitral valve.

Mitral valve stroke volume = 0.785 × (3.0 cm) squared ×
10 cm

= 71 cm cubed

Let's step outside the numbers again to make sure we got the numbers from the right place.

> You measured the mitral valve, where, the annulus or the tips of the leaflets?
>
> The annulus.
>
> Where do you measure the velocity?
>
> Same place. Get the stuff at the same place, not different places!
>
> Which kind of Doppler did you use?
>
> Pulsed wave, because we wanted a specific velocity at a specific place.

Calculation of Aortic Regurgitant Volume

Note well, young budding TEE'ogists. To calculate the aortic regurgitant volume, you must assume there is no mitral regurgitation going on either. Again, you need one equation, one unknown. Put in one equation and two unknowns, it won't work.

So, to the numbers:

> Regurgitant volume aortic valve + mitral valve stroke volume = LVOT SV

The ventricle is "loaded" with two volumes during regurgitation, the blood pouring backward from the incompetent aortic valve, and the blood flowing forward through the mitral valve. Then WHOOSH, both these volumes go blasting out the aortic valve.

> Regurgitant volume aortic valve + 71 ml = 94 ml
>
> Regurgitant volume AV = 94 ml – 71 ml
>
> = 23 ml

Still not convinced the mitral valve has to be competent? Let's load up the ventricle then WHOOSH it out both valves.

> Regurgitant volume AV + MV stroke volume = LVOT SV + MV regurgitant volume
>
> *Unknown* regurgitant volume + 71 ml = 23 ml + *unknown* MV regurgitant volume

No way, Jose. Too many unknowns.

Think about what's really happening in these problems. On the exam, they are sure to throw some kind of curve at you, so if you understand the physical reality of what's flowing where, you should handle it. If you think you can just "plug and forget," you'll get tripped up.

Calculation of Aortic Regurgitant Fraction

What amount of the total ejected blood ends up going backward?

Blood going backward/blood going forward = regurgitant fraction

Regurgitant volume aortic insufficiency/forward volume through LVOT = regurgitant fraction

23 ml/94 ml = 0.24 (or, by percentage, 24%)

Units check? (Do it every time) Yes. Common sense check? Yes.

Calculation of Aortic Regurgitant Orifice Area

Back to the cylinder of blood moving around. Get an area, multiply it by a length, and that gives you the volume of your cylinder of blood. Make sure the area and the velocity (recall that the velocity, when outlined, yields your TVI, or, length), are measured at the same place.

Aortic regurgitant orifice area × TVI aortic regurg = regurgitant volume AI

Think it through: you have an area (of regurg), a length (of regurg), and a volume (of regurg). It all makes sense, so now grind the numbers:

Aortic regurgitant orifice area × 160 cm = 23 cm cubed

= 23 cm cubed/160 cm

= 0.14 cm squared

Units? Good. Common sense? Um. That's pretty tiny for an aortic valve, but wait, this is the area where *regurgitation* is occurring, not the *entire* valve area. You can picture that this patient has an aortic dissection, so the aortic root is stretched, making the aortic valves not able to completely reach each other, and leaving a small area "uncovered" in the middle. Through that, 23 ml of blood per beat flows back into the heart. Then, yes, the aortic regurgitant orifice area of 0.14 cm squared makes sense.

Say you had come up with an aortic regurgitation orifice area of 1.2 cm squared. That would leave a gigantic gap. Blood would go like a house afire into the ventricle, giving an enormous regurgitant volume and, in all likelihood, a moribund patient.

Calculation of Cardiac Output

You are interested in what goes forward here. Regurgitant flow is not really output, it's "backward-put." So to calculate cardiac output, you need a real, live stroke volume that actually gets "out there," and as well you need a heart rate.

Cardiac output = 71 ml (the SV of the MV) × 80 bpm

= 5.6 L/m

Whoa! You say, wait just a darn tootin' minute here, partner, who said anything about the mitral valve? I thought, well, I thought we wanted cardiac output, like as in from the left ventricle out to the body. Who gives a damn about the "cardiac output" from the left atrium to the left ventricle?

Back to the continuity equation. We are talking about uninterrupted *forward* flow. The amount of blood that leaves the left atrium and doesn't come back (recall the mitral valve is OK), must be the amount that leaves the ventricle. As long as the forward flow is not diverted in its forward movement.

Look at flow in a different way to convince yourself that the continuity equation holds.

Pretend 71 ml of blood enters the left ventricle from the left atrium; then 71 ml do NOT go forward and out of the heart. Say only 50 ml goes out of the heart with each beat, and then 71 ml keeps entering the left ventricle through the mitral valve.

With each beat of the heart, the left ventricle gets 21 ml bigger. At the end of a minute, the heart will have 1600 ml of blood just hanging around, looking for a good time. At the end of the hour, your heart will be 96,000 ml bigger, or 96 L big. Echo findings in such a case would be remarkable, to say the least. Even the most vigorous patient might find handling such a volume load to be beyond his or her capacity.

Let's say you were given this problem and I said the patient had a VSD. Could the continuity equation come to the rescue? No. Do a sample problem to satisfy yourself of this.

Pretend that you magically know that 71 ml of blood enters through the mitral valve and 23 ml enters through regurgitation. That is, 71 ml of blood enters the left ventricle from the mitral valve, and 23 ml enters the left ventricle from regurgitant flow, so now the total ventricular volume of 94 ml goes WHOOSH! But how much goes out the aortic valve, and how much goes out the VSD? No way of knowing.

Calculation of Left Ventricular End-Diastolic Pressure

You'll have a high-pressure chamber, a choke point where a certain amount of pressure is lost, and a low-pressure area with the "leftover" pressure.

We're in diastole, so the ventricle is relaxing; that's the low-pressure area. The aorta just got a blast of blood, so there's high-pressure there. The choke point is the regurgitant valve. We can get the pressure from the measured velocity (using our old buddy, Bernoulli).

Aortic pressure in diastole (the high-pressure area) − the pressure lost in the choke point (the velocity of aortic regurg, which we'll use to get a pressure gradient by delta P = 4 × [velocity] squared; remember, velocity in meters/second to get pressure in mm Hg) = left ventricular end-diastolic pressure (the low-pressure area, and our unknown).

Now, to make it more mathematical and less wordy:

Systemic diastolic pressure − gradient across aortic valve
= LV EDP

60 mm Hg − 4 × (3 meters/second) squared = LV EDP

60 mm Hg − 36 mm Hg = LV EDP

LV EDP = 24 mm Hg

Units check? Check. Common sense check? Yes. Blood flowing into the left ventricle through regurgitation should create some pressure there. Nothing ridiculous. (Say you came up with an LV EDP of 130 mm Hg; that's higher than systolic pressure, and during diastole? No way.) So, this value satisfies the common sense test.

CASE 5 70-yo male with worsening dyspnea on exertion.

VITAL SIGNS

- Heart rate: 70 bpm
- Systemic BP: 100/50 mm Hg
- CVP: 12 mm Hg

TEE DATA

- LVOT diameter: 2.0 cm
- LVOT TVI: 20 cm
- MV TVI: 90 cm
- MV pressure half-time (PHT): 300 ms
- Peak trans-mitral end-diastolic velocity (EDV): 2 meters/second
- Pulmonary insufficiency EDV: 2.5 meters/second

CALCULATE

- Mitral valve area by pressure half-time
- Mitral valve area by continuity equation
- Pulmonary artery diastolic pressure

Calculation of Mitral Valve Area by Pressure Half-time

Area = 220/PHT

Where the hell did pressure half-time come from?

The rate of pressure (not velocity, but pressure) decline across the stenotic mitral valve orifice is determined by the cross-sectional area of the orifice. A tiny pinhole of a mitral valve would take a long time to empty. A totally normal, enormous mitral valve would allow the blood to fall through in no time flat. The picture tells the quantitative story.

The quantitative equation has been empirically worked out:

Area = 220/PHT

How? Doppler half-times were compared to cath lab studies, and this magic number appeared.

PRESSURE HALF TIME

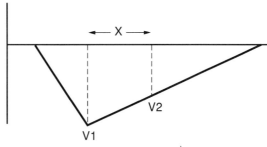

X = Time for *Pressure* to ↓ 50%

Draw a line down the E wave of mitral flow; make that line go right to 0. Ignore the A wave. Find the halfway point down the slope that corresponds to the *pressure* (recall, delta pressure = 4 × [velocity] squared); that is the halfway point. Do not go to the halfway point as far as *velocity* is concerned. As luck is with us, the computer on the TEE can do this.

So, back to the problem, what is the mitral valve area by PHT?

Area = 220/300 milliseconds

= 0.7 cm squared

Units check? Yes. If you use this equation, and use milliseconds, you get cm squared. Common sense? Yep. That's a tight mitral valve, and that goes along with the clinical picture of worsening dyspnea on exertion.

Calculation of Mitral Valve Area by Continuity Equation

So, we have a cylinder of blood in which we can measure the flow through our old friend, the LVOT:

Flow through LVOT = area of blood cylinder × length of blood cylinder

That, by continuity, must equal the flow through the mitral valve, so let's create that cylinder of blood:

Flow through mitral valve = area of mitral valve (our *unknown*) × length of that cylinder

Flow through mitral valve = area MV × TVI MV

If we believe in continuity, and, amen, amen, by now you *must* believe, then set the flow through the mitral valve equal to the flow through the LVOT:

Area MV × TVI MV = area LVOT × TVI LVOT

Area MV × 90 cm = 0.785 (2.0 cm) squared × 20 cm

Cross multiply and divide and you get

Area MV = 0.7 cm squared

Hot damn! Just like the pressure half-time way! Well bend me over an Adirondack chair and spank me with a two-by-four 'til I say "Mama!"

Calculation of Pulmonary Artery Diastolic Pressure

Remember, we're in diastole. Know where the high-pressure area, the choke point (where we'll get a gradient), and the low-pressure area with its "leftover" pressure are.

In diastole, the *high* pressure is in the *pulmonary artery*. It just received a blast of blood from the right ventricle. The *right ventricle*, in contrast, is *relaxing* after a hard day at the systole office. The *choke point* is the *pulmonary artery*, where blood is pouring back into the right ventricle.

High-pressure area: pulmonary artery

Choke point: pulmonic valve

Low-pressure area: right ventricle

PA diastolic pressure − choke point in pulmonic valve = RV EDP

Unknown − 4 × (2.5 meters/second) squared = RV EDP

Uh, er...Where is the RV EDP? Have we got one equation, two unknowns? I cry foul!

Hold on, professor. Let's find a good approximation of the RV EDP. How about the CVP? Well, think about it.

If there is no big pressure gradient between the right atrium and the right ventricle (there is no mention made of tricuspid stenosis), then, yes, in diastole, with the tricuspid valve open, the prevailing pressure in the right atrium should reflect the pressure in the right ventricle. So put 12 mm Hg into the right ventricle:

PA end-diastolic pressure − 4 × (2.5 meters/second) squared = 12 mm Hg

PA EDP = 25 mm Hg + 12 mm Hg

= 37 mm Hg

Satisfy yourself that the units and the common sense hold true.

CASE 6
54-yo man is having MV surgery. A-line, Swan, TEE. TEE shows thickened MV leaflets with diastolic doming and restricted opening. There is 2+ MR and no AI. You get the following:

VITAL SIGNS

- Heart rate: 100 bpm

- Systemic BP: 136/80 mm Hg

- Thermodilution cardiac output: 3.8 L/min

TEE DATA

- MV pressure half-time: 215 milliseconds

- Peak trans-mitral E velocity: 240 cm/second

- Mean trans-mitral velocity: 194 cm/second

- TVI mitral inflow: 55 cm

- TVI MR: 85 cm

- MS PISA radius: 1.4 cm

- PISA alias velocity: 30 cm/second

- MV alpha angle: 120 degrees

CALCULATE

- Peak trans-mitral pressure gradient

- Mitral valve area by pressure half-time

- Area of PISA

- Mitral valve area using PISA

- Mitral valve stroke volume

- Mitral valve regurgitant volume
- Mitral valve regurgitant fraction
- Effective MV regurgitant orifice area

Yipes. Killer.

Just start pounding, it'll unfold.

Calculation of Peak Trans-Mitral Pressure Gradient

OK, this is not the end of the world. We've used velocities to give us gradients before. The trusty old warhorse of Bernoulli comes trotting out.

Delta P = 4 × velocity squared

= 4 × (2.4 meters/second) squared

= 23 mm Hg

Note that they tried to fake you out by giving you the trans-mitral E velocity in cm/second. You need, in the Bernoulli equation, to have velocity in meters/second to get the answer in mm Hg. If you had said

Delta P = 4 × (240) squared

you would have ended up with a gradient of 57,600 mm Hg. If you see such a patient, DUCK, for his atrium is about to blow that wing of the hospital to smithereens.

Calculation of Mitral Valve Area by Pressure Half-time

Our new friend, area = 220/PHT, comes in here.

Area = 220/215 milliseconds

= 1.0 cm squared

Units OK? Yes. Common sense OK? Yes, this is a small mitral valve, which goes along with the TEE findings of diastolic doming and restricted opening. Just as an exercise, pretend he had a good mitral valve, one that opened right up and emptied real fast. What would you see?

A faster pressure half-time, say, 110 milliseconds to empty half way. And that means what? An area of 220/110, or 2 cm squared. A bigger valve. Faster emptying. Makes sense.

Calculation of Area of PISA

PISA area = 2 × pi × radius squared when the PISA hemisphere is flush and flat against the mitral valve. But when the PISA is at an angle to the mitral valve annulus plane, then the PISA area is less. The area of the PISA is then

PISA area = 2 × pi × radius squared × alpha angle/180

= 2 × pi × (1.4 cm) squared × 120/180

= 8.2 cm squared

If that angle is giving you trouble, consider two extreme examples to satisfy yourself that the angle does, indeed, decrease the area of the PISA hemisphere.

Consider 180 degrees; in other words, there is no angle. Then the "angle part" of the equation is 180/180 or 1. And the area is just that of a hemisphere,

2 × pi × radius squared

Consider 90 degrees. That looks like, and does, cut the area off by half.

Area = 2 × pi × radius squared × 90/180

= 2 × pi × radius squared × 0.5

Now consider a ridiculous angle, 0 degrees. That means there IS no PISA radius at all, and the area should be 0.

Area = 2 × pi × radius squared × 0/180

= 0

Calculation of Mitral Valve Area Using PISA

Um. Wait a minute here. Time and again, we've used the cylinder idea. You have an area; multiply it by a length (the TVI), and you get your stroke volume. The units work out right, common sense usually prevails, Ford's in his flivver, and all's right with the world.

But, er, we don't *have* a length measured in handy units of cm. Now we have an aliasing velocity in cm/second and a velocity of the mitral valve flow in cm/second. Well, wait, that *will* work out.

Area PISA × velocity (aliasing) will give us the volume/second going through the mitral valve. Well and good.

Area MV × velocity (MV peak) will give us the volume/second going through the mitral valve. By the grace of continuity, these amounts have to be the same. So we can set them equal to each other.

In earlier problems, we had set two cylinders of blood equal to each other (LVOT area × LVOT length = mitral valve area × mitral valve length). Now we have just taken it a step further by setting two *cylinders/second* equal to each other (PISA area × PISA velocity = mitral valve area × mitral valve velocity).

To review, then, this problem yields

Area PISA × velocity PISA = area MV (the *unknown*) × velocity MV
8.2 cm squared × 30 cm/second = area MV (the *unknown*) ×
240 cm/second

Cross multiply and divide and you get

Area MV = 1.0 cm squared

Holy consistency, Batman, the area turns out the same, even after all that work!

Calculation of Mitral Valve Stroke Volume

Things look a little more familiar here. Back to our "cylinder" of blood. No bothersome extra "/seconds" to worry about.

Area mitral valve × length mitral valve = stroke volume
mitral valve

Area MV × TVI MV = SV MV

1.0 cm squared × 55 cm = SV MV

SV MV = 55 ml

Units OK? Yes. Common sense OK? Yes: 55 ml is a decent stroke volume. Not super, but not ridiculously low or high.

Calculation of Mitral Valve Regurgitant Volume

Hubbada bubbada, what do we need to get this one? This does not jump off the page and drip obviousness.

OK, think about what's going on. Way back a hundred years ago you read that the patient has mitral regurg but no aortic insufficiency. So we load the left ventricle; where does the blood go?

There are only two "doors" into the left ventricle, the mitral valve pouring blood in during diastole, and, what else, how else could blood get in there? Blood could roll back into the left ventricle through the aortic valve. But no, look:

"There is 2+ MR but no AI."

"…no AI."

So, forget that. The only blood going into the left ventricle is the stroke volume passing the mitral valve, that is, the SV MV. That amount is 55 ml.

Now, what paths do we have OUT of the ventricle?

We still have the same two doors, the aortic and the mitral. Unlike during diastole, though, this time BOTH of the doors are open. The aortic valve functions its normal way, and pumps out a certain stroke volume, and the mitral valve is incompetent, so blood flows out that way too.

A ventricle filled with 55 ml divides its two exit pathways into two:

55 ml = volume out the aorta + volume out the mitral valve

But how much goes out the aorta? Where is our "usual" LVOT diameter and LVOT TVI? The bastards, they've left us high and dry.

Hold back your despair. It's time to go back, long ago, to a galaxy far, far away, where you used to figure stuff out *without* a TEE. Call this retro-cardio-technology.

You have a cardiac output, right, remember, from that Swan thing that they must have ordered from the Smithsonian? And you have a heart beat. (God, they probably actually felt a PULSE! How's that for a blast from the past? Why don't we all put on polyester leisure suits and head out to Studio 54?)

Cardiac output out the aorta = heart rate × stroke volume out the aorta

3.8 L/min = 100 beats/min × stroke volume out the aorta

Stroke volume out the aorta = 38 ml

So now we go back to what we were looking for:

55 ml (the amount loaded into the left ventricle) = 38 ml out the aorta + X ml out the incompetent mitral valve

55 ml = 38 ml + regurgitant volume

55 ml − 38 ml = regurgitant volume

Regurgitant volume = 17 ml

So, figuring this problem out was like the things every bride should wear, "*Something old, something new, something borrowed,* something blue, and a penny in her shoe."

Only without the blue and penny stuff.

Calculation of Mitral Valve Regurgitant Fraction

Nothing earth-shattering here:

Regurgitant fraction = regurgitant volume/total volume sent through MV

Regurgitant fraction = 17 ml/55 ml

Regurgitant fraction = 0.31, or, as a percentage, 31%

Units, common sense? Yeah, yeah, yeah. When will this chapter ever end?

Calculation of Effective MV Regurgitant Orifice Area

Cylinderville:

Area of regurgitation through the MV × length of regurg = volume of regurg

MV regurgitant area (the *unknown*) × TVI MV regurg = regurgitant volume MV

MV regurgitant area × 85 cm = 17 ml

MV regurgitant area = 17 ml/85 cm

= 0.2 cm squared

Makes sense, right units, so rock on. If this is starting to get repetitive, that is fine and dandy, sugar candy. These should be so drilled into you that you should be able to do these problems standing on your head. There are only a few ideas (move a cylinder of blood; know which way the blood is flowing; continuity; Bernoulli; area × length = volume; high-pressure area loses pressure in a gradient, which goes to the low-pressure area). And, no matter how the question is phrased, you get back to the same principles. If you go through the nine problems from their workshop, and understand how you got everything, you should ace this part of the test.

And if not, well hell, there's always next year.

CASE 7   56-yo man presents for AV surgery.

VITAL SIGNS

- Heart rate: 84 bpm
- Systemic BP: 90/70 mm Hg
- CVP: 14 mm Hg
- BSA: 1.98 meters squared

TEE DATA

- LVOT TVI
- LVOT diameter
- Aortic valve mean gradient
- Aortic valve TVI
- TR peak velocity

CALCULATE

- LVOT stroke volume
- Cardiac output and index
- Aortic valve area
- Pulmonary artery systolic pressure

No kidding, by now you should be able to nail this stuff.

Calculation of LVOT Stroke Volume

Move the cylinder, move the cylinder, move the cylinder of blood.

Stroke volume out the LVOT = area of LVOT × length (the TVI)

SV LVOT = 0.785 × (diameter LVOT) squared × 23 cm

= 0.785 × (2.2 cm) squared × 23 cm

= 87 ml

which makes sense in terms of both units and normal physiology.

Calculation of Cardiac Output and Index

Puh-leeze! After jumping through the flaming hoops of PISA alpha angles, this is downright pedestrian.

Cardiac output = stroke volume × TVI

Cardiac output = 87 ml × 23 cm

Cardiac output = 1951 cm to the 4th power

Units, um. Common sense, er… HEY, WAIT A MINUTE! Aha, so you see, you can fall asleep at the wheel here and just grab any old number and plug it in. Then, when your numbers and units come out phony baloney, the klaxons should start clanging.

Cardiac output = stroke volume × heart rate

CO = 87 ml/heartbeat × 84 heartbeats/minute

= 7.3 L/minute

That's more like it. That unit makes sense, and an output of 7.3 L/minute you've seen before in the OR.

Cardiac index = CO/BSA

CI = 7.3 L/minute/1.98 meters squared

= 3.7 L/minute/meter squared

Calculation of Aortic Valve Area

Continuity equation, here we come. The cylinder of blood going out the LVOT = the cylinder of blood going out the aortic valve. We already have the cylinder of LVOT blood.

LVOT SV (the cylinder of blood we calculated first) = area of the aortic valve (unbeknownst to us at present, but soon to yield to our astute powers of calculation) × length (TVI of the aortic valve)

87 ml = area of AV × 122 cm

Cross multiply to get

Area of AV = 87 ml/122 cm

= 0.7 cm squared

Right units, right size for a fellow with aortic stenosis.

Calculation of Pulmonary Artery Systolic Pressure

Go with the concept of finding the high-pressure area, finding the choke point where you lose pressure across a gradient, and the leftover low-pressure area.

In systole, the right ventricle is the high-pressure area, and the right ventricle is squeezing into the pulmonary artery. So, hmm, but they gave us tricuspid valve regurg values and velocities.

Damn.

That's, sort of, going the wrong way. Hmm. Think, think, think, like Winnie the Pooh does.

We want to find the pulmonary artery pressure, darn the luck, but we seem "at a remove" from what we want to find out. So we'll have to approach this from a more intellectual point of view.

The pulmonic valve, so we are given to understand, is OK, no stenosis there. So, whatever pressure the right ventricle generates should go right into the pulmonary artery. There is no "choke point" causing a gradient loss.

That's a start. The pulmonary artery systolic pressure will be the right ventricular systolic pressure. Can we figure *that* out?

Yes! We are no longer "at a remove" from useful information. We have our high-pressure area, our "choke point" where we lose pressure across a gradient, and our low-pressure area.

RV pressure – pressure lost across the tricuspid valve gradient = low-pressure area in the right atrium (the CVP)

RV P – 4 × (3.6 meters/second) squared = 14 mm Hg

RV P – 52 mm Hg = 14 mm Hg

RV P = 66 mm Hg

Right units, makes sense that a right ventricle might have to generate a lot of pressure in the face of a diseased heart. (He has a tight aortic valve plus tricuspid regurg. Ay caramba! You think *you've* got problems.)

And, to answer the question, since the RV generates 66 mm Hg, and the pulmonic valve has no stenosis, then it makes sense that the pulmonary artery "sees" all that pressure and thus the PA systolic pressure is 66 mm Hg.

You CAN figure these things out, even when it's not super obvious!

CASE 8   78-yo man undergoing AAA surgery becomes hypoxic and hypotensive with cross-clamping of the abdominal aorta. TEE reveals 1+ to 2+ MR, 1+ TR without AS or AI.

VITAL SIGNS

- Heart rate: 110 bpm
- Systemic BP: 85/50 mm Hg
- CVP: 8 mm Hg

TEE DATA

- Aortic valve side: 2.3 cm
- Aortic valve TVI: 12 cm
- Peak velocity MR: 3.5 meters/second
- Peak velocity TR: 3.5 meters/second

CALCULATE

- Aortic valve area
- Stroke volume

- Cardiac output
- Left atrial pressure

Calculation of Aortic Valve Area

What's with the *side* schtick? I got the cylinder thing down like nuthin', and now we got, what, Euclidean geometry, come on!

Chill. Like Avril Lavigne says in her song, "It's all been done before."

We have to turn ourselves in knots and avoid planimetry when the aortic valve is *diseased*. Plane old (pardon the pun) planimetry can't nail the aortic valve area when the valve is all calcified, bumpy, irregular, and grotty mundo. But hark, the case states the patient is "without AS or AI," so it turns out we *can* use planimetry.

Just when you had it all figured out, they throw in a *normal* one to screw you up.

Call the aortic valve area an equilateral triangle, solve for the area of said triangle, and you come up with

Area = 0.433 × (side) squared

Area of this aortic valve = 0.433 × (2.3 cm) squared

= 2.3 cm squared

Units make sense, and, wonder of wonders, the common sense works too, because 2.3 cm squared is within the normal range. That jibes with "without AS or AI."

Calculation of Stroke Volume

Roll that cylinder, er, well, call it a kind of "triangular cylinder"? Either way, the area of the blood × the length (TVI) of the blood will give us a volume, however triangular we may envision it.

Area of AV × TVI = stroke volume

2.3 cm squared × 12 cm = SV

SV = 28 ml

Units work out, and common sense, ... whoa Nelly. Stroke volume of 28 ml. Not exactly irrational exuberance on the part of the heart is it. Does that make clinical sense?

A 28-ml stroke volume is Bad News Bears Breaking Training. But look at the overall picture — hypoxemic, hypotensive, old patient, just had the aorta cross-clamped. Them's a lot of reasons to be doing poorly. So, yes, this result, though alarming, does satisfy the "common sense" criterion.

Calculation of Cardiac Output

I won't try to fake you out twice.

Stroke volume × heart rate = CO

29 ml × 110 bpm = 3.2 L/minute

Bad, which goes along with the clinical picture.

Calculation of Left Atrial Pressure

Where is the high-pressure area? The left ventricle.

Where is the choke point? The mitral valve.

Where is the low-pressure area? The left atrium.

The left ventricle, with its systolic pressure, loses pressure (use Bernoulli) across the mitral valve, which then lands in the left atrium.

LV systolic pressure − 4 × (3.5 meters/second) squared = left atrial pressure 85 mm Hg (the systemic blood pressure, since the left ventricle creates the pressure and goes out a nonstenotic aortic valve into the systemic circulation) − 49 mm Hg = left atrial pressure

85 mm Hg − 49 mm Hg = left atrial pressure

Left atrial pressure = 36 mm Hg

Crikey (as the Croc Hunter says), this patient is overloaded and doing badly. If things don't get better soon, he may go Down Under.

CASE 9   81-yo woman develops severe dyspnea and a harsh systolic murmur 8 days after an acute MI. She gets intubated and rolls into an ICU near you. Stat TEE shows a VSD with left-to-right shunting. Aortic and mitral valves are normal.

VITAL SIGNS

- Heart rate: 100 bpm
- Systemic BP: 100/60 mm Hg

TEE DATA

- LVOT diameter: 1.8 cm
- LVOT TVI: 17 cm
- PA diameter: 2.4 cm
- PA TVI: 22 cm
- VSD peak velocity: 3.2 meters/second

CALCULATE

- LVOT stroke volume
- Cardiac output
- Pulmonary artery stroke volume
- Pulmonary artery blood flow
- Shunt fraction (Qp/Qs)
- Peak right ventricular systolic pressure

Calculation of LVOT Stroke Volume

Volume = area × distance (just in case you forgot, or in case you were abducted by a UFO and had your brains sucked out)

Volume through LVOT = area of LVOT × length (TVI) of the LVOT

SV = 0.785 × diameter squared × 17 cm

= 0.785 × (1.8 cm) squared × 17 cm

= 43 ml

Any hesitation on embracing this? Just the usual stuff, right? But what about the VSD, does that gum things up? Remember, whatever may be happening in the septum is *below* you. You measured the LVOT, which is 5 to 10 mm below the aortic valve. That area is real, and the TVI you measured with your precisely placed pulsed-wave Doppler is real. That LVOT flow is the blood that has escaped whatever carnage is happening at the ventricular septum. LVOT blood made good its escape from the left ventricle.

Calculation of Cardiac Output

Remember the anatomy; you can do the simple

Cardiac output out the LVOT = heart rate × stroke volume of the LVOT

Don't sweat the VSD, you got past that, no worries, mate.

CO = heart rate × SV

CO = 100 bpm × 43 ml = 4.3 L/minute

Good units, good common sense.

Calculation of Pulmonary Artery Stroke Volume

Just sit back, relax, and let the cylinder of blood flow.

Area of PA (0.785 × diameter squared) × TVI PA (22 cm) = PA SV

PA SV = 99 ml

Right units. Now, that stroke volume looks a little larger than the stroke volume we just calculated for the blood going out the LVOT into the systemic circulation. Good Golly Miss Molly, has the inviolable truth of the continuity equation been undone? Has the world gone mad?

The horror. The horror.

But wait, hope springs eternal. Remember, the continuity equation holds ONLY IF the flow is uninterrupted. And we have an interruption here, a VSD! We have another exit door out of the left ventricle.

Given that, then, this answer *does* make common sense.

Calculation of Pulmonary Artery Blood Flow

PA SV × heart rate = total flow through the PA

99 ml/heartbeat × 100 bpm = PA blood flow

PA blood flow = 9.9 L/minute

Units, good. Common sense? That's a lot of blood zipping through the PA. But then, if the right side is getting its "normal flow" (say 5 L/minute or so), plus a blast from the left side coming across the VSD (recall that the history mentions an MI with development of a VSD with left-to-right shunting), then 9.9 L/minute does make common sense.

Calculation of Shunt Fraction (Qp/Qs)

Shunt fraction compares pulmonary flow to systemic flow.

Qp/Qs = 9.9 L/minute / 4.3 L/minute

= 2.3

No units, that works. More blood going through the pulmonary vasculature than the systemic? Yes, that makes sense because the high-pressure left side is squishing over to the low-pressure right side, "shorting" the systemic blood flow and augmenting the pulmonary blood flow.

Calculation of Peak Right Ventricular Systolic Pressure

Where is the high-pressure chamber? The left ventricle. Since there is no aortic stenosis, the systolic pressure in the left ventricle is all conveyed to the aorta. So we can take the systemic pressure as our left ventricular pressure.

Where is the choke point, across which the high-pressure area loses pressure? The VSD. Bernoulli will tell us the pressure drop.

Where is the low-pressure point? The right ventricle. (Our unknown.)

LV systolic pressure − 4 × (3.2 meters/second) squared = RV systolic pressure

100 mm Hg − 41 mm Hg = RV systolic pressure

RV systolic pressure = 59 mm Hg

And that, in so many words, is that. You are now a bona fide Hemodynamo-Doc.

Epilogue: Smooth Sailing

"Nothing ever happens on my voyages."

EDWARD SMITH
Captain of the Titanic

There you have it. TEE in a nutshell.

Now, whether you decide to make TEE a part of your OR, ER, or ICU practice, I wish you smooth sailing, just like Captain Smith had. (At least for the first half of his trip.)

If you decide to take the PTEeXAM, best of luck.

I hope this simplified introduction helped to clarify a point or two about the groovalacious world of transesophageal echocardiography.

See you under a bridge somewhere!

Chris Gallagher
February 25, 2004

Index